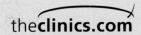

PET CLINICS

Infection and Inflammation

Guest Editors
ABASS ALAVI, MD
HONGMING ZHUANG, MD, PhD

April 2006 • Volume 1 • Number 2

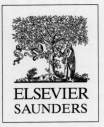

ELSEVIER
SAUNDERS

An imprint of Elsevier, Inc
PHILADELPHIA LONDON TORONTO MONTREAL SYDNEY TOKYO

W.B. SAUNDERS COMPANY

A Division of Elsevier Inc.

1600 John F. Kennedy Boulevard • Suite 1800 • Philadelphia, Pennsylvania 19103-2899

http://www.theclinics.com

PET CLINICS Volume 1, Number 2
April 2006 ISSN 1556-8598, ISBN 1-4160-3730-6

Editor: Barton Dudlick

PET Clinics (ISSN 1556-8598) is published quarterly by W.B. Saunders, 360 Park Avenue South, New York, NY 10010-1710. Months of publication are January, April, July, and October. Business and Editorial Offices: 1600 John F. Kennedy Blvd., Suite 1800, Philadelphia, PA 19103-2899. Accounting and Circulation Offices: 6277 Sea Harbor Drive, Orlando, FL 32887-4800. Periodicals postage paid at New York, NY, and additional mailing offices. Subscription prices are USD 150 per year for US individuals, USD 210 per year for US institutions, USD 75 per year for US students and residents, USD 170 per year for Canadian individuals, USD 200 per year for Canadian institutions, USD 170 per year for international individuals, USD 230 per year for international institutions and USD 85 per year for Canadian and foreign students/residents. To receive student and resident rate, orders must be accompanied by name of affiliated institution, date of term, and the signature of program/residency coordinator on institution letterhead. Orders will be billed at individual rate until proof of status is received. Foreign air speed delivery is included in all Clinics subscription prices. All prices are subject to change without notice. POSTMASTER: Send address changes to *PET Clinics*, Elsevier Periodicals Customer Service, 6277 Sea Harbor Drive, Orlando, FL 32887-4800. **Customer Service: 1-800-654-2452 (US). From outside of the US, call (+1) 407-345-4000.**

Printed in the United States of America.

INFECTION AND INFLAMMATION

EWALD KRESNIK, MD
Department of Nuclear Medicine and
Endocrinology, PET/CT Centre, General Hospital,
Klagenfurt, Austria

RAKESH KUMAR, MD
Associate Professor, Department of Nuclear
Medicine, All India Institute of Medical Sciences,
New Delhi, India

TORSTEN LIERSCH, MD
Department of General Surgery, University of
Göttingen, Göttingen, Germany

PETER LIND, MD
Department of Nuclear Medicine and
Endocrinology, PET/CT Centre, General Hospital,
Klagenfurt, Austria

MICHEL G. MALAISE, MD, PhD
Head, Division of Rheumatology, University
Hospital of Liège, University of Liège, Center of
Cell and Molecular Therapy, Liège, Belgium

AYSE MAVI, MD
Research Fellow, Department of Radiology,
Hospital of the University of Pennsylvania,
Philadelphia, Pennsylvania

JOHANNES MELLER, MD
Adjunct Professor and Director, Department of
Nuclear Medicine, University of Göttingen,
Göttingen, Germany

PETER MIKOSCH, MD
Department of Internal Medicine and
Gastroenterology, General Hospital,
Klagenfurt, Austria

CARSTEN OLIVER SAHLMANN, MD
Department of Nuclear Medicine,
University of Göttingen,
Göttingen, Germany

PETER HAO TANG, BA
Research Coordinator, Division of Nuclear
Medicine, Department of Radiology,
Hospital of the University of Pennsylvania,
Philadelphia, Pennsylvania

MARTIN A. WALTER, MD
Institute of Nuclear Medicine,
University Hospital Basel,
Basel, Switzerland

HUA YANG, MD
Division of Nuclear Medicine,
Department of Radiology,
University of Pennsylvania
School of Medicine, Hospital of the
University of Pennsylvania,
Philadelphia, Pennsylvania

JIAN Q. YU, MD
Director of Nuclear Medicine/Positron Emission
Tomography; Associate Member,
Division of Medical Science,
Department of Diagnostic Imaging,
Fox Chase Cancer Center,
Philadelphia, Pennsylvania

HONGMING ZHUANG, MD, PhD
Chief, Division of Nuclear Medicine,
The Children's Hospital of Philadelphia;
and Assistant Professor, Department of Radiology,
University of Pennsylvania School of Medicine,
Philadelphia, Pennsylvania

INFECTION AND INFLAMMATION

Volume 1 • Number 2 • April 2006

Contents

Preface   xi

Abass Alavi and Hongming Zhuang

Critical Role of 18F-Labeled Fluorodeoxyglucose PET in the Management of Patients with Arthroplasty   99

Hongming Zhuang, Hua Yang, and Abass Alavi

The most frequent complications after arthroplasty are aseptic loosening and infection. It is often difficult to differentiate aseptic loosening from infection. The management of these two distinct clinical identities is quite different, however. Treatment of aseptic loosening usually requires one-step revision surgery, whereas treatment of infection requires antimicrobial therapy for an extended period before inserting a new prosthesis. Infection associated with arthroplasty is a serious complication and should be treated adequately before proceeding with a surgical intervention. PET with 18F-labeled fluorodeoxyglucose (FDG) has been proposed as an accurate technique for evaluating painful arthroplasty. This review addresses the applications of FDG-PET in such clinical settings. In addition, the potential of PET in the assessing the viability of bone grafts in revision arthroplasty is discussed.

Nonprosthesis Orthopedic Applications of ^{18}F Fluoro-2-Deoxy-D-Glucose PET in the Detection of Osteomyelitis   107

Johannes Meller, Carsten Oliver Sahlmann, Torsten Liersch, Peter Hao Tang, and Abass Alavi

This article describes the impact of [^{18}F]2-fluoro-2-deoxy-D-glucose (FDG) PET in the diagnosis of non–prosthesis-related orthopedic infections and inflammation. FDG-PET has an excellent sensitivity in the detection of osteomyelitis (OM). Early data indicate that FDG-PET may be more specific than MRI in diagnosing OM. The role of the combination of FDG and PET-CT in the diagnosis of OM is likely to be determined as this combination is used on a routine basis. Early data from studies in rheumatoid arthritis indicate that FDG-PET is highly accurate in early diagnosis and that it provides results comparable to the most advanced conventional techniques.

Application of 18F-Fluorodeoxyglucose and PET in Evaluation of the Diabetic Foot   123

John Hochhold, Hua Yang, Hongming Zhuang, and Abass Alavi

Diagnosing acute and chronic osteomyelitis in the diabetic foot remains a challenge for health care providers. The timely and accurate diagnosis of osteomyelitis has an impact on clinical management of the diabetic foot. Widely used conventional modalities used to noninvasively assess osteomyelitis in the diabetic foot include radiography, MRI, triple-phase bone scintigraphy, and 111-indium–labeled leukocyte imaging. These radiographic and scintigraphic techniques have significant shortcomings. 18F-fluorodeoxyglucose (FDG) PET is increasingly used for the diagnosis of a variety of infectious and inflammatory processes. FDG-PET is an optimal modality for a timely and accurate diagnosis of osteomyelitis as well as for distinguishing it from other pathologic disorders in superficial and deep tissue structures in diabetic patients with a neuropathic foot. This powerful technique is likely to demonstrate greater levels of accuracy than conventional modalities in assessing this complex clinical problem.

PET Imaging of Arthritis   131

Roland Hustinx and Michel G. Malaise

Fluorodeoxyglucose (FDG) PET imaging of arthritis is still in its infancy. Neither the optimal methodology nor the real clinical value is known at this time. Nevertheless, initial results are highly encouraging and the feasibility of the technique is demonstrated. PET findings are correlated with results obtained with state-of-the-art MRI and ultrasonography as well as with established clinical assessment of rheumatoid arthritis. There are indications that FDG-PET may provide unique information regarding the prognosis and early response to treatment. The mechanism of FDG uptake in the diseased joints has to be clarified further, but the available data indicate that it is well suited for imaging inflammatory joint disorders and, possibly, osteoarthritis. What lies ahead is the important work of clinical validation to verify the diagnostic and prognostic accuracy before envisioning a clinical role in routine practice.

Evaluating the Role of Fluorodeoxyglucose PET Imaging in the Management of Patients with Sarcoidosis   141

Jian Q. Yu, Hongming Zhuang, Ayse Mavi, and Abass Alavi

Sarcoidosis as a distinct disease entity was introduced more than 100 years ago. Most patients are asymptomatic and are never diagnosed, but a segment of the affected population is detected by incidental findings. The signs and symptoms of the disease are nonspecific, and this poses a challenge for accurate diagnosis. Along with many clinical specialties that take part in managing these patients, imaging techniques are playing an increasingly important role in the diagnosis, determining the extent of the disease, monitoring the response to therapy, and detecting recurrence. This article briefly describes the role of the existing diagnostic imaging studies, including plain radiography, CT, MRI, and conventional nuclear medicine imaging studies, in this disease entity. The major emphasis is placed on PET, however, as a new and exciting modality for assessing inflammatory diseases. This review discusses the utility of 18F-fluorodeoxyglucose PET in assessing disease activity at various anatomic sites, including the lungs, heart, central nervous system, and other organs.

Role of Fluorodeoxyglucose PET in Inflammatory Bowel Disease: A Review   153

Ewald Kresnik, Peter Mikosch, Hans-Juergen Gallowitsch, Susanne Kohlfürst, Isabell Igerc, and Peter Lind

Inflammatory bowel disease (IBD) requires a complex diagnostic workup. In contrast to endoscopy and cross-sectional imaging methods, scintigraphy enables a complete survey of the whole small and large bowel intestinal tract with a single noninvasive examination. For detection of IBD, 80% to 90% sensitivity and 92% to 100% specificity can be found for conventional scintigraphy. A new imaging method like fluorine-18 (F-18) fluorodeoxyglucose PET has been shown to be useful in tumor diagnostics. An increased tracer uptake in PET can also be found in several inflammatory disorders. A major problem in PET is the limited anatomic information and nonspecific tracer uptake within the colon, however, which may lead to false-positive results. New imaging methods like combined PET/CT can help to solve the problem, because physiologic tracer uptake can be easily distinguished from pathologic lesions as a result of the anatomic detail provided by CT.

Value of 18-Fluoro-2-Deoxyglucose PET in the Management of Patients with Fever of Unknown Origin   163

Ghassan El-Haddad, Abass Alavi, and Hongming Zhuang

Timely identification of the cause of fever of unknown origin (FUO) is crucial for patient management. The initial evaluation for FUO includes a thorough history, physical examination, and standard laboratory and imaging tests. Advanced diagnostic imaging modalities, such as CT, MRI, and standard nuclear medicine procedures, are commonly used for the assessment of these patients. This article reviews different diagnostic imaging studies that are currently used for examining patients with FUO but also focuses on the role of 18-fluoro-2-deoxyglucose positron emission tomography and its impact on the management of patients with FUO.

[^{18}F]Fluorodeoxyglucose PET in Large Vessel Vasculitis   179

Martin A. Walter

[^{18}F]fluorodeoxyglucose (FDG) PET is a noninvasive metabolic imaging modality based on the regional distribution of [^{18}F]FDG that is highly effective in assessing the activity and extent of giant cell arteritis and Takayasu's arteritis, respectively. Metabolic imaging using [^{18}F]FDG-PET has been shown to identify more affected vascular regions than morphologic imaging with MRI in both diseases. The visual grading of vascular [^{18}F]FDG uptake helps to discriminate arteritis from atherosclerosis and therefore provides high specificity. High sensitivity is attained by scanning during the active inflammatory phase. Thus, [^{18}F]FDG-PET has the potential to develop into a valuable tool in the diagnostic workup of giant cell arteritis and Takayasu's arteritis.

Assessment of Therapy Response by Fluorine-18 Fluorodeoxyglucose PET in Infection and Inflammation   191

Rakesh Kumar, Anil Chauhan, Hongming Zhuang, and Abass Alavi

PET has been extremely useful in evaluating the treatment response to chemotherapy or radiotherapy in patients with various neoplastic disorders. Little is known about the clinical usefulness of fluorine-18 fluorodeoxyglucose (FDG) PET for assessing the treatment response, however, and few studies have been described in patients with inflammatory or infectious diseases. Most of the studies demonstrate a definite role of FDG-PET in the diagnosis and evaluation of the treatment response and disease activity in patients with vasculitis. In other inflammatory or infectious diseases, only a few studies with a limited number of patients have been published. Nevertheless, if we extrapolate the use of PET in inflammatory or infectious diseases, it can be assumed that PET may hold a promising future role in the follow-up of inflammatory or infectious diseases.

Index   **199**

FORTHCOMING ISSUES

July 2006

Lymphomas
Ora Israel, MD, *Guest Editor*

October 2006

Lung Cancer
James Fletcher, MD, *Guest Editor*

RECENT ISSUE

January 2006

Breast Cancer
Norbert Avril, MD, *Guest Editor*

PET CLINICS APRIL 2006

GOAL STATEMENT

The goal of the *PET Clinics* is to keep practicing radiologists and radiology residents up to date with current clinical practice in positron emission tomography by providing timely articles reviewing the state-of-the-art in patient care.

ACCREDITATION

PET Clinics is planned and implemented in accordance with the Essential Areas and Policies of the Accreditation Council for Continuing Medical Education (ACCME) through the joint sponsorship of the University of Virginia School of Medicine and Elsevier. The University of Virginia School of Medicine is accredited by the ACCME to provide continuing medical education for physicians.

The University of Virginia School of Medicine designates this educational activity for a maximum of 60 category 1 credits per year, 15 category 1 credits per issue, toward the AMA Physician's Recognition Award. Each physician should claim only those credits that he/she actually spent in the activity.

The American Medical Association has determined that physicians not licensed in the US who participate in this CME activity are eligible for AMA PRA category 1 credit.

Category 1 credit can be earned by reading the text material, taking the CME examination online at http://www.theclinics.com/home/cme, and completing the evaluation. After taking the test, you will be required to review any and all incorrect answers. Following completion of the test and evaluation, your credit will be awarded and you may print your certificate.

FACULTY DISCLOSURE/CONFLICT OF INTEREST

The University of Virginia School of Medicine, as an ACCME accredited provider, endorses and strives to comply with the Accreditation Council for Continuing Medical Education (ACCME) Standards of Commercial Support, Commonwealth of Virginia statutes, University of Virginia policies and procedures, and associated federal and private regulations and guidelines on the need for disclosure and monitoring of proprietary and financial interests that may affect the scientific integrity and balance of content delivered in continuing medical education activities under our auspices.

The University of Virginia School of Medicine requires that all CME activities accredited through this institution be developed independently and be scientifically rigorous, balanced and objective in the presentation/discussion of its content, theories and practices.

All authors/editors participating in an accredited CME activity are expected to disclose to the readers relevant financial relationships with commercial entities occurring within the past 12 months (such as grants or research support, employee, consultant, stock holder, member of speakers bureau, etc.). The University of Virginia School of Medicine will employ appropriate mechanisms to resolve potential conflicts of interest to maintain the standards of fair and balanced education to the reader. Questions about specific strategies can be directed to the Office of Continuing Medical Education, University of Virginia School of Medicine, Charlottesville, Virginia.

The authors/editors listed below have identified no professional or financial affiliations for themselves or their spouse/partner: Abass Alavi, MD, Editorial Board; Anil Chauhan, MD; Barton Dudlick, Acquisitions Editor; Ghassan El-Haddad, MD; Hans Juergen Gallowitsch, MD; Peter Hao Tang, BA; Johannes Hochhold, MD; Roland Hustinx, MD, PhD; Isabell Igerc, MD; Susanne Kohlfurst, MD; Ewald Kresnik, MD; Rakesh Kumar, MD; Torsten Liersch, MD; Peter Lind, MD; Michel G. Malaise, MD, PhD; Ayse Mavi, MD; Johannes Meller, MD; Carolyn Cidis Meltzer, MD, Editorial Board; Peter Mikosch, MD; Patrice K. Rehm, MD, Editorial Board; Carter Oliver Sahlmann, MD; Peter H. Tang, BA; Martin A. Walter, MD; Hua Yang, MD; Jian Q. Yu, MD; and, Hongming Zhuang, MD, PhD.

The authors/editors listed below identified the following professional or financial affiliations for themselves or their spouse/partner:

Disclosure of Discussion of non-FDA approved uses for pharmaceutical products and/or medical devices:
The University of Virginia School of Medicine, as an ACCME provider, requires that all faculty presenters identify and disclose any "off label" uses for pharmaceutical and medical device products. The University of Virginia School of Medicine recommends that each physician fully review all the available data on new products or procedures prior to instituting them with patients.

TO ENROLL

To enroll in the *PET Clinics* Continuing Medical Education program, call customer service at 1-800-654-2452 or visit us online at www.theclinics.com/home/cme. The CME program is available to subscribers for an additional fee of $175.00.

POSITRON
EMISSION
TOMOGRAPHY

PET Clin 1 (2006) xi–xvi

Preface
^{18}F-Fluorodeoxyglucose PET Imaging: An Ideal Technique for Assessing Inflammation and Infection

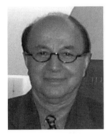

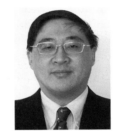

Abass Alavi, MD   Hongming Zhuang, MD, PhD
                Guest Editors

Abass Alavi, MD
Division of Nuclear Medicine
Department of Radiology
University of Pennsylvania School of Medicine
Hospital of the University of Pennsylvania
110 Donner Building
3400 Spruce Street
Philadelphia, PA 19104, USA

E-mail address:
abass.alavi@uphs.upenn.edu

Hongming Zhuang, MD, PhD
Division of Nuclear Medicine
Department of Radiology
University of Pennsylvania School of Medicine
The Children's Hospital of Philadelphia
Philadelphia, PA 19104, USA

E-mail address:
Zhuang@email.chop.edu

Early diagnosis or exclusion of infection and inflammation is of the utmost importance for the optimal management of patients with such common disorders. Although in certain settings, this diagnosis can be made without any difficulty, in most others, the attending clinicians may encounter substantial challenges in detecting and locating the exact site of the pathologic processes. Modern imaging techniques, such as CT and MRI, provide excellent structural resolution for visualizing advanced diseases, including those related to infection and inflammation disorders. These modalities are of limited value in detecting early disease, however, regardless of the cause. Therefore, functional and metabolic imaging techniques are often needed to complement the role of anatomic imaging techniques in most clinical settings.

Over the past 3 decades, we have witnessed the introduction of several scintigraphic techniques, especially labeled leukocyte imaging, for examining

doi:10.1016/j.cpet.2006.04.008

patients with suspected infection or inflammation [1–3]. Unfortunately, these procedures suffer from substantial shortcomings. These procedures are time-consuming, labor-intensive, and costly. In addition, results may not available for at least 24 hours, which may delay optimal treatment for most patients. The conventional planar imaging techniques that are used for these techniques also suffer from poor special resolution, and thus fail to pinpoint the exact location of the affected sites. In addition, the sensitivity of these methods is relatively low. Furthermore, detection of infection and inflammation in certain locations, such as skeletal structures with significant red marrow activity, is quite difficult. Also, there are concerns about the safety of these preparations because of the potential for contamination from hepatitis virus and other pathogens [4]. Radiolabeled antibody, which was introduced recently for detecting sites of infection, was withdrawn from market because of serious side effects. Therefore, there is a great desire to use a methodology that may overcome many of the difficulties encountered.

In spite of great successes achieved by ^{18}F-fluorodeoxyglucose (FDG) PET imaging in the evaluation of malignant disorders, the test is not specific for cancer, and this has affected its performance in certain anatomic sites and after therapeutic interventions. Soon after the introduction of FDG-PET for human studies, it was noted that lesions with substantial inflammatory cells also appear positive on FDG-PET. Reviewing the literature indicated that the activated inflammatory cells, such as macrophages, have significantly increased glycolysis [5–9]. In addition, multiple cytokines are released at the sites of infection and inflammation, which further increases glycolysis in the inflammatory cells. Also, the number of glucose transporters on the surface of inflammatory cells is increased, which further enhances uptake of FDG in tissues that contain these cells. Therefore, on FDG-PET images, sites of infection or noninfectious inflammation may be indistinguishable from those of malignant disease. Also, it has been shown that malignant tissues contain a large number of inflammatory cells; therefore, a fraction of uptake in such tissues could be attributed to increased glycolysis in these cells [10].

Obviously, uptake of FDG in nonmalignant tissues posses a challenge in a setting in which the presence and characterization of suspected or proven cancer is of clinical concern. The role of this technique could be further enhanced in situations in which infection and inflammation are the foci of the investigation, however. These initial observations and incidental repots in the literature eventually led to the systematic assessment of the value of FDG-PET imaging in the settings in which the presence of infection or inflammation poses a clinical challenge. Early experience at the University of Pennsylvania and some European institutions has demonstrated that FDG-PET is quite sensitive for detecting infection in complicated orthopedic conditions [11–14]. Animal experiments further clarified the phenomenon of increased glycolysis in the inflamed tissues under controlled conditions [15–18]. These animal studies demonstrated the superiority of FDG-PET compared with other nuclear medicine techniques for this purpose.

Major indications for ^{18}F-fluorodeoxyglucose PET

Chronic osteomyelitis

As a result of altered bony structures attributable to trauma, surgery, and other interventions, the accurate diagnosis of chronic osteomyelitis is often difficult with existing radiologic or nuclear medicine techniques. Although the use of radiolabeled white blood cells (WBCs) in combination with bone marrow scans has been reported to be highly accurate for the detection of chronic osteomyelitis, the role of these techniques is limited in most clinical settings.

MRI is quite accurate in diagnosing infections in anatomically intact bone structures, but in patients who have undergone surgical intervention, this technique is unable to distinguish between nonspecific edema and chronic infection. Other tests, such as that for erythrocyte sedimentation rate (ESR) and C-reactive proteins, are also insensitive and nonspecific in detecting chronic osteomyelitis. FDG-PET has been shown to be highly sensitive for the detection of chronic osteomyelitis even in patients who have been treated with antibiotics before they undergo FDG-PET imaging [11,19]. This is in contrast to WBC imaging, where the sensitivity is significantly affected by prior use of antibiotics. Also, tomographic images provided by PET allow generation of images with excellent spatial resolution that can be coregistered and compared with anatomic images, such as CT and MRI, for precise localization of infection. Several publications in the literature have demonstrated the superiority of FDG-PET over imaging with radiolabeled WBCs with an accuracy exceeding 90% in this clinical setting [11,19,20]. Therefore, FDG-PET seems to be the study of choice when chronic osteomyelitis is suspected. This is particularly true when this type of infection is suspected in the axial skeleton or anywhere with a significant concentration of red marrow. In contrast to bone scintigraphy, which remains positive for an extended period after fracture [21], FDG uptake normalizes in less than 2 to

3 months after such accidents [22,23]. This reduces many of the false-positive results when osteomyelitis is suspected in complicated fractures.

Infected prosthesis

With the increased life expectancy in developed and developing countries around the world, a large number of patients with degenerative hip and knee joint diseases are receiving artificial prostheses for this disabling condition. This is particularly true for the hip joint, for which more than 300,000 patients undergo arthroplasty in United States every year. Although 10% of these patients experience significant pain, only 1% are found to have periprosthetic infection after the initial operation. The remaining patients are found to have loosening without infection. The incidence of infection increases substantially after the second or third operation. Differentiation between these two conditions has become a major challenge to practicing orthopedic surgeons. Although revising the prosthesis cures aseptic loosening alone, superimposed infection would require intensive treatment before revision surgery is undertaken. Various nuclear medicine techniques, including radiolabeled leukocyte scans and sulfur colloid bone marrow scans, and bone scintigraphy have been used for differentiating between these two conditions [24–27]. Unfortunately, none of the current imaging techniques combined with joint aspirations can make this distinction with high accuracy. Several reports in the literature have demonstrated the high sensitivity and specificity of FDG-PET for assessing these patients [28–30]. Based on the data from the University of Pennsylvania and other centers, a specific pattern for infection has been defined when infection is proven at the site. This includes the presence of FDG uptake between the bone and the prosthesis in the midshaft portion of the prosthesis for hip implantation in these patients. In the literature, the accuracy of this technique using the criteria described previously exceeds 90% as reported by several groups. Interestingly, frequently, some degree of inflammation is noted around the neck, which is almost entirely noninfectious in nature and has no clinical relevance [31]. The role of FDG-PET in assessing knee infection is somewhat limited because of the suboptimal specificity of the technique compared with a hip prosthesis. Further research should be performed to define the role of FDG-PET in the latter group.

Fever of unknown origin

Fever of unknown origin (FUO) is caused by numerous underlying causes, including infections, noninfectious inflammation, and a variety of malignancies. The accurate localization and characterization of the underlying cause of FUO should certainly improve the management of these patients. Usually, many of these patients experience the disabling effects of the disease for an extended period, and current imaging techniques have a low yield in detecting and characterizing the cause of this disorder. The current techniques, including anatomic imaging modalities, radiolabeled WBC imaging, and gallium-67 citrate scintigraphy, have a relatively low yield in this population. In contrast, FDG-PET scanning allows for the identification of inflammatory and malignant disorders as the underlying cause in most patients. FDG-PET has been shown to detect pathologic processes that were not detected with conventional nuclear medicine techniques [32–35]. Also, results from PET are available within 1 to 2 hours compared with 2 to 3 days with the conventional techniques. Therefore, FDG-PET imaging may prove to be the modality of choice in patients with FUO.

Vasculitis

Vasculitis is a group of multiple different disorders characterized by accumulation of leukocytes in the blood vessel walls, which results in reactive damage in mural structure. These disorders are primarily classified based on the thickness of the involved vessels. Many authors have supported the role of FDG-PET for early diagnosis and assessment of the response to therapy in patients with several types of vasculitis [36–40]. Almost all studies have demonstrated a definite role for FDG-PET in establishing the diagnosis, defining the extent of the disease, determining treatment response, and detecting disease activity in patients with vasculitis. In three studies that included 20 patients who underwent baseline and follow-up imaging studies, FDG-PET results were compared with those of MRI for the diagnosis and evaluation of response to treatment [38–40]. These studies demonstrated that FDG-PET and MRI are effective noninvasive techniques for detecting early vasculitis; however, FDG-PET was noted to be superior to MRI in demonstrating disease activity after treatment during the follow-up period.

Inflammatory bowel disease

Physiologic FDG uptake in the bowel varies considerably with regard to its anatomic distribution and intensity; therefore, detection of inflammatory bowel disease (IBD) with this technique poses a challenge in most patients. A few studies have demonstrated the usefulness of FDG-PET in detecting disease activity in patients with suspected IBD [41–45]. In our experience, physiologic FDG uptake in the bowel is dependent on many factors. Age is probably the most important factor for FDG uptake, and the intensity and extent of its activity are substantial in older subjects. Therefore, FDG-PET is likely to be useful in the pediatric population for early diagnosis, assessing the extent of the disease, and evaluating treatment response and disease activity in various stages of the disease. A good correlation has been demonstrated between the degree of inflammation and the uptake of FDG-labeled WBCs [45].

Lung and pleural diseases

Occupational lung diseases, such as pneumoconiosis, asbestosis, and silicosis, are incurable lung disorders, because these conditions are usually diagnosed in the late stages when therapeutic intervention may not be effective. FDG-PET may be useful in the early diagnosis of these often debilitating diseases. There are several reports demonstrating increased FDG lung uptake in these patients [46,47]. The increased FDG lung uptake is likely attributable to activated fibroblasts and inflammatory cells at the diseased sites. Asbestos-related lung and pleural diseases could be benign or malignant in nature. It is important to differentiate between these two conditions. Several studies have shown the superiority of FDG-PET over CT in determining malignant transformation of reactive pleural diseases [48,49].

Atherosclerosis

It is well documented that inflammation is an integral part of atherosclerosis. Studies from our laboratory as well as others have shown that inflammatory cells, predominantly macrophages, take up FDG in atherosclerotic plaques [50]. Therefore, a functional imaging modality like FDG PET can detect and localize inflammatory changes in the arterial wall representing early stages of atherosclerosis [51]. Baller and colleagues [52] demonstrated improvement in coronary flow reserve as determined by PET after 6 months of cholesterol-lowering therapy in patients with early stages of coronary atherosclerosis. Therefore, we believe that FDG-PET may play an important role in assessing the effects of cholesterol-lowering therapy noninvasively by visualizing the degree of FDG uptake of this tracer in the aortic wall.

Other possible applications

FDG-PET has been shown to have a high sensitivity in early infection in vascular grafts. Also, FDG-PET seems to make a distinction between toxoplasmosis from lymphoma as complications of AIDS. Although lymphoma seems to be active with PET, toxoplasmosis is relatively negative with this technique. The role of FDG in investigating the diabetic foot is under investigation in several centers around the world, and early data indicate that PET is sensitive and specific in diagnosing osteomyelitis and distinguishing it from superimposed skin ulceration. FDG-PET may prove to be of value in detecting clots in blood vessels [53–57].

References

[1] Bennink RJ, Peeters M, Rutgeerts P, et al. Evaluation of early treatment response and predicting the need for colectomy in active ulcerative colitis with 99mTc-HMPAO white blood cell scintigraphy. J Nucl Med 2004;45:1698–704.

[2] Stokkel MP, Reigman HE, Pauwels EK. Scintigraphic head-to-head comparison between 99mTc-WBCs and 99mTc-LeukoScan in the evaluation of inflammatory bowel disease: a pilot study. Eur J Nucl Med Mol Imaging 2002;29:251–4.

[3] Termaat MF, Raijmakers PG, Scholten HJ, et al. The accuracy of diagnostic imaging for the assessment of chronic osteomyelitis: a systematic review and meta-analysis. J Bone Joint Surg Am 2005;87:2464–71.

[4] Rojas-Burke J. Health officials reacting to infection mishaps. J Nucl Med 1992;33:13N–27N.

[5] Chakrabarti R, Jung CY, Lee TP, et al. Changes in glucose-transport and transporter isoforms during the activation of human peripheral blood lymphocytes by phytohemagglutinin. J Immunol 1994;152:2660–8.

[6] Sorbara LR, Maldarelli F, Chamoun G, et al. Human immunodeficiency virus type 1 infection of H9 cells induces increased glucose transporter expression. J Virol 1996;70:7275–9.

[7] Yamada S, Kubota K, Kubota R, et al. High accumulation of fluorine-18-fluorodeoxyglucose in turpentine-induced inflammatory tissue. J Nucl Med 1995;36:1301–6.

[8] Miyamoto M, Sato EF, Nishikawa M, et al. Effect of endogenously generated nitric oxide on the energy metabolism of peritoneal macrophages. Physiol Chem Phys Med NMR 2003;35:1–11.

[9] Kawaguchi T, Veech RL, Uyeda K. Regulation of energy metabolism in macrophages during hypoxia. Roles of fructose 2,6-bisphosphate and ribose 1,5-bisphosphate. J Biol Chem 2001;276:28554–61.

[10] Kubota R, Yamada S, Kubota K, et al. Intratumoral distribution of fluorine-18-fluorodeoxyglucose in vivo—high accumulation in macrophages and granulation tissues studied by microautoradiograph. J Nucl Med 1992;33:1972–80.

[11] De Winter F, Van de Wiele C, Vogelaers D, et al. Fluorine-18 fluorodeoxyglucose-positron emission tomography: a highly accurate imaging modality for the diagnosis of chronic musculoskeletal infections. J Bone Joint Surg Am 2001;83:651–60.

[12] Meller J, Koster G, Liersch T, et al. Chronic bacterial osteomyelitis: prospective comparison of F-18-FDG imaging with a dual-head coincidence camera and In-111-labelled autologous leucocyte scintigraphy. Eur J Nucl Med 2002;29:53–60.

[13] Zhuang H, Duarte PS, Pourdehand M, et al. Exclusion of chronic osteomyelitis with F-18 fluorodeoxyglucose positron emission tomographic imaging. Clin Nucl Med 2000;25:281–4.

[14] Zhuang H, Alavi A. 18-Fluorodeoxyglucose positron emission tomographic imaging in the detection and monitoring of infection and inflammation. Semin Nucl Med 2002;32:47–59.

[15] Koort JK, Makinen TJ, Knuuti J, et al. Comparative F-18-FDG PET of experimental Staphylococcus aureus osteomyelitis and normal bone healing. J Nucl Med 2004;45:1406–11.

[16] Zhuang H, Pourdehnad M, Lambright ES, et al. Dual time point F-18-FDG PET imaging for differentiating malignant from inflammatory processes. J Nucl Med 2001;42:1412–7.

[17] Jones-Jackson L, Walker R, Purnell G, et al. Early detection of bone infection and differentiation from post-surgical inflammation using 2-deoxy-2-[(18)F]-fluoro-d-glucose positron emission tomography (FDG-PET) in an animal model. J Orthop Res 2005;23:1484–9.

[18] Sahlmann CO, Siefker U, Lehmann K, et al. Dual time point 2- F-18 fluoro-2'-deoxyglucose positron emission tomography in chronic bacterial osteomyelitis. Nucl Med Commun 2004;25:819–23.

[19] Guhlmann A, Brecht-Krauss D, Suger G, et al. Fluorine-18-FDG PET and technetium-99m antigranulocyte antibody scintigraphy in chronic osteomyelitis. J Nucl Med 1998;39:2145–52.

[20] Kalicke T, Schmitz A, Risse JH, et al. Fluorine-18 fluorodeoxyglucose PET in infectious bone diseases: results of histologically confirmed cases. Eur J Nucl Med 2000;27:524–8.

[21] Matin P. Appearance of bone scans following fractures, including immediate and long-term studies. J Nucl Med 1979;20:1227–31.

[22] Schmitz A, Risse JH, Textor J, et al. FDG-PET findings of vertebral compression fractures in osteoporosis: preliminary results. Osteoporos Int 2002;13:755–61.

[23] Zhuang H, Sam JW, Chacko TK, et al. Rapid normalization of osseous FDG uptake following traumatic or surgical fractures. Eur J Nucl Med Mol Imaging 2003;30:1096–103.

[24] Scher DM, Pak K, Lonner JH, et al. The predictive value of indium-111 leukocyte scans in the diagnosis of infected total hip, knee, or resection arthroplasties. J Arthroplasty 2000;15:295–300.

[25] Palestro CJ, Kim CK, Swyer AJ, et al. Total-hip arthroplasty: periprosthetic indium-111 labeled leukocyte activity and complementary technetium-99m-sulfur colloid imaging in suspected infection. J Nucl Med 1990;31:1950–4.

[26] Joseph TN, Mujtaba M, Chen AL, et al. Efficacy of combined technetium-99m sulfur colloid/indium-111 leukocyte scans to detect infected total hip and knee arthroplasties. J Arthroplasty 2001;16:753–8.

[27] Kraemer WJ, Saplys R, Waddell JP, et al. Bone scan, gallium scan, and hip aspiration in the diagnosis of infected total hip arthroplasty. J Arthroplasty 1993;8:611–6.

[28] Reinartz P, Mumme T, Hermanns B, et al. Radionuclide imaging of the painful hip arthroplasty. J Bone Joint Surg Br 2005;87:465–70.

[29] Mumme T, Reinartz P, Alfer J, et al. Diagnostic values of positron emission tomography versus triple-phase bone scan in hip arthroplasty loosening. Arch Orthop Trauma Surg 2005;125:322–9.

[30] Zhuang H, Duarte PS, Pourdehnad M, et al. The promising role of F-18-FDG PET in detecting infected lower limb prosthesis implants. J Nucl Med 2001;42:44–8.

[31] Zhuang H, Chacko TK, Hickeson M, et al. Persistent non-specific FDG uptake on PET imaging following hip arthroplasty. Eur J Nucl Med Mol Imaging 2002;29:1328–33.

[32] Meller J, Altenvoerde G, Lehmann K, et al. Fever of unknown origin—prospective comparison of 18 FDG-imaging with a double head coincidence camera (DHCC) and Ga-67 citrate SPECT. Eur J Nucl Med 2001;28:OS387.

[33] Dadparvar S, Anderson GS, Bhargava P, et al. Paraneoplastic encephalitis associated with cystic teratoma is detected by fluorodeoxyglucose positron emission tomography with negative magnetic resonance image findings. Clin Nucl Med 2003;28:893–6.

[34] Xiu Y, Yu JQ, Cheng E, et al. Sarcoidosis demonstrated by FDG PET imaging with negative findings on gallium scintigraphy. Clin Nucl Med 2005;30:193–5.

[35] Blockmans D, Knockaert D, Maes A, et al. Clinical value of [F-18]fluoro-deoxyglucose positron emission tomography for patients with fever of unknown origin. Clin Infect Dis 2001;32:191–6.

[36] Brodmann M, Lipp RW, Passath A, et al. The role of 2-F-18-fluoro-2-deoxy-D-glucose positron emission tomography in the diagnosis of giant cell arteritis of the temporal arteries. Rheumatol 2004;43:241–2.

[37] Meller J, Strutz F, Siefker J, et al. Early diagnosis and follow-up of aortitis with F-18 FDG PET and MRI. Eur J Nucl Med Mol Imaging 2003;30:730–6.

[38] Moreno D, Yuste JR, Rodriguez M, et al. Positron emission tomography use in the diagnosis and follow up of Takayasu's arteritis. Ann Rheum Dis 2005;64:1091–3.

[39] Scheel AK, Meller J, Vosshenrich R, et al. Diagnosis and follow up of aortitis in the elderly. Ann Rheum Dis 2004;63:1507–10.

[40] Andrews J, Al-Nahhas A, Pennell DJ, et al. Noninvasive imaging in the diagnosis and management of Takayasu's arteritis. Ann Rheum Dis 2004;63:995–1000.

[41] Bicik I, Bauerfeind P, Breitbach T, et al. Inflammatory bowel disease activity measured by positron-emission tomography. Lancet 1997;350:262.

[42] Kresnik E, Mikosch P, Gallowitsch HJ, et al. F-18 fluorodeoxyglucose positron emission tomogra-

phy in the diagnosis of inflammatory bowel disease. Clin Nucl Med 2001;26:867.

[43] Vehling D, Neurath M, Siessmeier T, et al. FDG-PET, anti-granulocyte-scintigraphy and hydro-MRI in the determination of bowel wall inflammation in Crohn's disease [abstract]. J Nucl Med 2000;41:11P.

[44] Jacobson K, Mernagh JR, Green T, et al. Positron emission tomography in the investigation of pediatric inflammatory bowel disease [abstract]. Gastroenterology 1999;116:A742.

[45] Pio B, Byrne F, Aranda R, et al. Noninvasive quantification of bowel inflammation through positron emission tomography imaging of 2-deoxy-2-[18F]fluoro-D-glucose-labeled white blood cells. Mol Imaging Biol 2003;5:271–7.

[46] Strauss LG. Fluorine-18 deoxyglucose and false-positive results: a major problem in the diagnostics of oncological patients. Eur J Nucl Med 1996;23:1409–15.

[47] Cook GJR, Maisey MN, Fogelman I. Normal variants, artefacts and interpretative pitfalls in PET imaging with 18-fluoro-2-deoxyglucose and carbon-11 methionine. Eur J Nucl Med 1999;26: 1363–78.

[48] Gerbaudo VH, Sugarbaker DJ, Britz-Cunningham S, et al. Assessment of malignant pleural mesothelioma with F-18-FDG dual-head gamma-camera coincidence imaging: comparison with histopathology. J Nucl Med 2002;43:1144–9.

[49] Balogova S, Grahek D, Kerrou K, et al. [18F]-FDG imaging in apparently isolated pleural lesions. Rev Pneumol Clin 2003;59:275–88.

[50] El-Haddad G, Zhuang H, Gupta N, et al. Evolving role of positron emission tomography in the management of patients with inflammatory and other benign disorders. Semin Nucl Med 2004; 34:313–29.

[51] Rudd JHF, Warburton EA, Fryer TD, et al. Imaging atherosclerotic plaque inflammation with F-18-fluorodeoxyglucose positron emission tomography. Circulation 2002;105:2708–11.

[52] Baller D, Notohamiprodjo G, Gleichmann U, et al. Improvement in coronary flow reserve determined by positron emission tomography after 6 months of cholesterol-lowering therapy in patients with early stages of coronary atherosclerosis. Circulation 1999;99:2871–5.

[53] Miceli M, Atoui R, Walker R, et al. Diagnosis of deep septic thrombophlebitis in cancer patients by fluorine-18 fluorodeoxyglucose positron emission tomography scanning: a preliminary report. J Clin Oncol 2004;22:1949–56.

[54] Bhargava P, Kumar R, Zhuang H, et al. Catheter-related focal FDG activity on whole body PET imaging. Clin Nucl Med 2004;29:238–42.

[55] Chang KJ, Zhuang H, Alavi A. Detection of chronic recurrent lower extremity deep venous thrombosis on fluorine-18 fluorodeoxyglucose positron emission tomography. Clin Nucl Med 2000;25:838–9.

[56] Kikuchi M, Yamamoto E, Shiomi Y, et al. Internal and external jugular vein thrombosis with marked accumulation of FDG. Br J Radiol 2004; 77:888–90.

[57] Siosteen AK, Celsing F, Jacobsson H. FDG uptake in a catheter-related thrombus simulating relapse of lymphoma. Clin Nucl Med 2005;30:338–9.

POSITRON
EMISSION
TOMOGRAPHY

PET Clin 1 (2006) 99–106

ELSEVIER
SAUNDERS

Critical Role of 18F-Labeled Fluorodeoxyglucose PET in the Management of Patients with Arthroplasty

Hongming Zhuang, MD, PhD[a,b], Hua Yang, MD[a],
Abass Alavi, MD[a,*]

- Accuracy of 18F-labeled fluorodeoxyglucose PET in the evaluation of infection associated with arthroplasty with a dedicated full-ring PET scanner
- Potential sources of suboptimal results for fluorodeoxyglucose PET imaging in painful arthroplasty

- *Coincident camera*
- *Combined PET and CT*
- Evaluating bone allograft after hip revision arthroplasty
- Summary
- References

The success of arthroplasty has greatly improved the quality of life for many patients with degenerative, arthritic, or injured joints. Some patients develop persistent pain at the site of arthroplasty after surgery, however. In most patients, the pain is caused by biomechanical failure (loosening), whereas in a small number of such patients, it is attributable to periprosthetic infection [1–5]. One of the most difficult diagnostic challenges in patients with painful prostheses is how to distinguish between aseptic mechanical loosening and periprosthetic infection. Most periprosthetic infections remain undiagnosed before revision surgery is undertaken. Clinically, these two clinical entities have similar presentations. The current tests to establish the diagnosis of infection before surgery include routine radiography, bacterial culture after joint aspiration, three-phase bone scan, gallium scan, and labeled leukocyte scintigraphy. Results from these tests are suboptimal, however, because of high rates of false-positive and false-negative findings. Accurate diagnosis or exclusion of infection is critical before revision surgery. Treatment of aseptic loosening requires a single revision operation, whereas patients with infection require a long period of treatment before surgery is contemplated. Currently, multiple tests are used for differentiating aseptic loosening from infection. A white blood cell count, erythrocyte sedimentation rate, and C-reactive protein level are all frequently per-

This article is partially supported by an N14 grant 5R01AR048241 (to AA).
[a] Division of Nuclear Medicine, Department of Radiology, University of Pennsylvania School of Medicine, Hospital of the University of Pennsylvania, 110 Donner Building, 3400 Spruce Street, Philadelphia, PA 19104, USA
[b] Division of Nuclear Medicine, Department of Radiology, University of Pennsylvania School of Medicine, The Children's Hospital of Philadelphia, 34th Street and Civic Center Boulevard, Philadelphia, PA 19104, USA
* Corresponding author.
E-mail address: abass.alavi@uphs.upenn.edu (A. Alavi).

doi:10.1016/j.cpet.2006.01.001

formed for this purpose but provide nonspecific results. Plain films have a limited role in such clinical settings, because infection and loosening have similar findings. Aspiration biopsy, if positive, can confirm infection before surgery. A negative joint aspiration result cannot exclude the diagnosis of infection [6], however, especially in patients who have received antibiotic therapy before aspiration biopsy [7,8]. Bone and gallium scintigraphy was initially used in the evaluation of infection after arthroplasty. Most infections cannot be diagnosed accurately by bone and gallium scans, however [9]. Although three-phase bone scintigraphy has been used in the evaluation of painful prosthesis replacement, it lacks adequate accuracy [10]. Indium 111–labeled leukocyte scintigraphy, when combined with technetium (Tc)-99m–sulfur colloid bone marrow imaging, may provide reasonable accuracy for the detection of infection after arthroplasty [11–14]. This technique requires separating, labeling, and reinjection of the patient's white blood cells, however, which is quite complex and time-consuming and increases the chance of iatrogenic errors [15]. In addition, 24-hour delayed imaging is necessary before a diagnosis can be made, which further adds to the complexity of the procedure.

In recent years, 18F-labeled fluorodeoxyglucose (FDG) PET has been used successfully for assessing a multitude of malignant disorders. FDG is specific for neoplastic tumor, however, and it also accumulates at the sites of infection and inflammation [16–23]. As a result of these observations, FDG-PET has emerged as a promising imaging modality for the evaluation of a variety of infectious and inflammatory processes [24,25], including those of the musculoskeletal system [26–36]. There are reports indicating that FDG-PET is more accurate than conventional nuclear medicine procedures in the evaluation of inflammation or infection [37–39]. In addition to providing high-quality images within a reasonably short time, FDG-PET scan results are not adversely affected by a metal prosthesis [40]. Therefore, FDG-PET is emerging as an important imaging modality in the evaluation of arthroplasty-associated complications.

Accuracy of 18F-labeled fluorodeoxyglucose PET in the evaluation of infection associated with arthroplasty with a dedicated full-ring PET scanner

The accuracy of FDG-PET from the pooled data of the major publications in the English literature is 90.4% (range: 68.6%–100%) for assessing painful hip prostheses and 83.1% (range: 77.8%–100%) for knee prostheses [Table 1]. In general, most publications demonstrate that for the evaluation of possible hip prosthesis infection, the specificity of FDG-PET is slightly higher than its sensitivity. In contrast, FDG-PET has high sensitivity but moderate specificity for examining painful knee prostheses for infection [see Table 1].

The largest sample of patients with hip prostheses examined with FDG-PET was reported in a recent publication by Reinartz and colleagues [10]. In this study, these investigators recruited 63 patients with 92 hip prostheses with possible periprosthetic infection. They noted that the sensitivity, specificity, and accuracy of FDG-PET were 93.9%, 94.9%, and 94.6%, respectively. These results are in contrast to the results of three-phase bone scintigraphy, which achieved sensitivity, specificity, and accuracy of 68%, 76%, and 74%, respectively. The authors concluded that FDG-PET is a highly

Table 1: Accuracy of 18F-labeled fluorodeoxyglucose imaging of painful prostheses using a full-ring dedicated PET scanner

Type	Authors [reference]	Year	No. prostheses	Sensitivity	Specificity	Accuracy
Hip	Manthey et al [55]	2002	14	100% (3/3)	100% (11/11)	100% (14/14)
	Vanquickenborne et al [43]	2003	17	87.5% (7/8)	77.8% (7/9)	82.4% (14/17)
	Stumpe et al [44]	2004	35	33.3% (3/9)	80.8% (21/26)	68.6% (24/35)
	Reddy et al [42]	2005	81	91.3% (21/23)	96.5% (56/58)	95.1% (77/81)
	Reinartz et al [10]	2005	92	93.9% (31/33)	94.9% (56/59)	94.6% (87/92)
Hip total			239	85.5% (65/76)	92.6% (151/163)	90.4% (216/239)
Knee	Van Acker et al [53]	2001	21	100 (6/6)	73.3 (11/15)	81.0% (17/21)
	Zhuang et al [41]	2001	36	90.9% (10/11)	72.0% (18/25)	77.8% (28/36)
	Manthey et al [55]	2002	14	100% (1/1)	100% (13/13)	100% (14/14)
Knee Total			71	94.4% (17/18)	79.2% (42/53)	83.1% (59/71)

accurate diagnostic procedure that is able to differentiate reliably between aseptic loosening and periprosthetic infection [10]. The results of this investigation are similar to those of our group. In an early investigation by our group involving 62 patients and 74 lower extremity prostheses (36 knee and 38 hip prostheses), FDG-PET demonstrated an overall sensitivity of 90.5% and specificity of 81.1% in the diagnosis of periprosthetic infection [41]. The sensitivity, specificity, and accuracy of PET for detecting infection associated with 38 hip arthroplasties were 90%, 89.3%, and 89.5%, respectively [41]. In our group's recent data on 81 painful hip prostheses, FDG-PET correctly diagnosed 21 of the 23 infected cases, with a sensitivity of 91.3%. The results of FDG-PET were positive only in 2 of the 58 aseptic prostheses, with a specificity of 96.5%. FDG-PET imaging demonstrated a positive predictive value of 91.3% and a negative predictive value of 96.6%. The overall accuracy of FDG-PET in this clinical setting is 95.1% [42]. In certain studies with a small sample of patients, however, relatively low rates of accurate results have been reported. For example, in an investigation involving 17 hip prostheses, Vanquickenborne and coworkers [43] found that FDG-PET had a sensitivity of 87.5%, a specificity of 77.8%, and an accuracy of 82.4%. These results seem suboptimal compared with those of single photon emission computed tomography (SPECT) images with ^{99m}Tc-hexamethylpropyleneamine oxime (HMPAO)–labeled leukocyte scintigraphy. The least accurate result was reported by Stumpe and colleagues [44] when they showed that FDG-PET only has an accuracy of 68.6%.

Several factors might account for the discrepant results reported by the different groups. The first and probably most important answer for this variance is the lack of uniform criteria used for the diagnosis of periprosthetic infection. By now, it is well known that there is frequently nonspecific FDG uptake after hip arthroplasty, which can last as long as 2 decades in patients without any complications [45]. The nonspecific FDG activity is usually around the head and neck portion of the prosthesis [Fig. 1]. The nonspecific activity around the neck portion of the hip prosthesis is probably caused by the accumulation of macrophages and multinuclear giant cells attributable to polyethylene wear particles [46–48]. Therefore, caution should be exercised in interpreting FDG activity in these locations so as to minimize the number of false-positive results. In addition, the sites of the increased FDG accumulation seem to be more important than the intensity of the FDG uptake at these locations [49]. Vanquickenborne and colleagues [43] interpreted PET images to represent

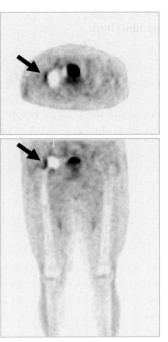

Fig. 1. Transaxial (*upper*) and coronal (*lower*) views of FDG-PET images of an asymptomatic patient with a history of right hip arthroplasty. Arrows point to the nonspecific FDG uptake in the neck region of the prosthesis.

infection when FDG uptake around the prosthesis is two scores higher than that in the contralateral distal femur. In contrast, Reinartz and his coworkers [10,50] considered infection as the diagnosis when increased FDG activity in the periprosthetic soft tissue and arthroplasty interface was observed. Our group [49,51] has used similar criteria for infection as those of Reinartz and his coworkers [10,50]. We think that the abnormal FDG uptake along the prosthesis-bone interface in the middle portion of the shaft of the prosthesis is the most reliable indicator of periprosthetic infection [Fig. 2]. The degree of FDG uptake alone can be misleading, because there is a significant overlap between aseptic loosening and periprosthetic infection with regard to the intensity of the activity noted on these scans [10]. In an investigation by Reinartz and colleagues [10] involving a total of 92 hip prostheses, the average standardized uptake value was 5.3 ± 2.7 for periprosthetic infection, which was not significantly different ($P = .35$) from that (5.0 ± 3.0) of aseptic loosening. This might explain why Vanquickenborne and coworkers [43] reported slightly less accurate results compared with those of the Reinartz and colleagues [10], because intensity of the activity was considered the major criterion used by former group for diagnosing

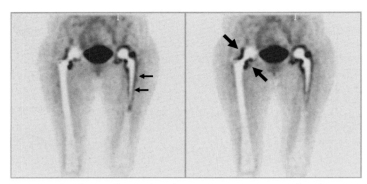

Fig. 2. A 59-year-old man with bilateral hip arthroplasty and pain on the left side. FDG-PET images revealed intense activity in the region of the neck of the right hip prosthesis (*large arrows*), which was interpreted to be a nonspecific finding and not representing infection. FDG-PET also demonstrated diffuse activity along the middle portion of the shaft of the left hip prosthesis (*small arrows*), which was considered strongly suggestive of periprosthetic infection. The periprosthetic infection was confirmed by subsequent surgery.

periprosthetic infection. In addition to different diagnostic criteria used by different groups, standards by which the presence of or lack of infection was confirmed and the composition of the patient population recruited, which included subjects with different prevalence of the disease, might also have contributed to the differences in the accuracy of the results reported by different investigators.

The experience with FDG-PET in the evaluation of knee prostheses is considerably less than that in hip prostheses. The accuracy of FDG-PET in the evaluation of knee prostheses is somewhat lower than that in hip prostheses [41] for unclear reasons. Capsulitis or synovitis attributable to the loosening of the knee prosthesis can result in intense FDG activity [52,53] that is difficult to distinguish from the hypermetabolism caused by infection. In addition, it has been proposed that attenuation correction–induced artifact around a knee prosthesis might render the interpretation difficult [54]. Van Acker and coworkers [53] assessed the potential of FDG-PET in a group of 21 patients with painful knee prostheses. Using focal FDG uptake at the bone-prosthesis interface as the criterion for infection, they found that the sensitivity, specificity, and positive predictive value of FDG-PET were 100%, 73%, and 60%, respectively, in the diagnosis of periprosthetic knee infection. Similarly, in a study involving 36 knee prostheses, the sensitivity, specificity, and positive predictive value of FDG-PET were shown to be 90.9%, 72.0%, and 58.8%, respectively [41]. In an investigation involving 14 painful knee prostheses evaluated by FDG-PET, however, Manthey and colleagues [55] were able to exclude infection in all the noninfected patients with sensitivity, specificity, and positive predictive values of 100%, 100%, and 100%, respectively. The number of patients in this investigation is relatively small; therefore, the results cannot be generalized

to the overall patient population referred for this examination. Also, similar to what was described for hip prostheses, different diagnostic criteria used by different groups could have contributed to the difference in the accuracy of the results reported by different groups.

Potential sources of suboptimal results for fluorodeoxyglucose PET imaging in painful arthroplasty

Coincident camera

It is important to note that evaluation of a painful prosthesis by a coincidence PET camera is likely to provide unsatisfactory results. Love and coworkers [56] studied FDG uptake in 40 hip and 19 knee prostheses using a coincidence detection system. They noted that regardless of the how the images were interpreted, the accuracy of this approach is suboptimal. The best accuracy by using the most favorable schemes was 71% (78% for hip prostheses and 58% for knee prostheses). In contrast, the accuracy of the combined leukocyte and bone marrow imaging was 95% in their study population. Therefore, the authors concluded that the coincidence detection system is less accurate than combined labeled leukocyte and bone marrow imaging for diagnosing infection of the failed prosthetic joint [56].

Combined PET and CT

The combined PET and CT instruments have certain advantages over PET alone in the evaluation of a variety of malignancies. Nevertheless, it is important to note that in contrast to conventional PET scanners, when a cesium (Cs)-137 or Germanium-68 (Ge-68) source is used for attenuation correction and is not significantly affected by metal [40,57,58], the

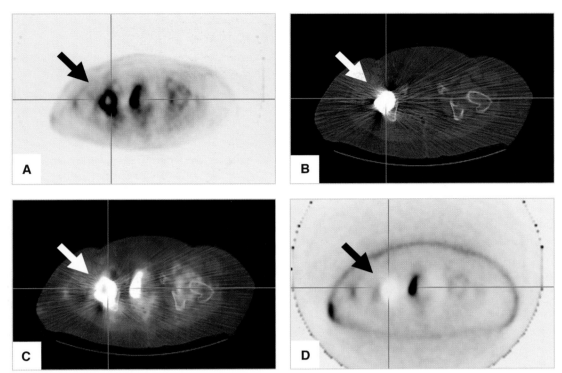

Fig. 3. PET-CT images from a patient with a right hip prosthesis. The attenuation-corrected image (*A*) demonstrated intense activity (*black arrow*) corresponding to the metal prosthesis on CT (*B*) and fused PET-CT (*C*) images (*white arrows*). This intense activity is an artifact caused by CT for reconstructing attenuation correction imaging. (*D*) Non–attenuation-corrected image is negative in the corresponding region (*black arrow*).

CT-corrected images often have significant artifact at the location of the prosthesis, which interferes with the optimal interpretation of the result generated [Fig. 3] [59,60]. Therefore, when PET-CT is used for the evaluation of a painful prosthesis, non–attenuation-corrected images must be interpreted for this purpose so as to avoid false-positive results.

Evaluating bone allograft after hip revision arthroplasty

Bone loss with or without evidence of aseptic loosening or periprosthetic infection is a long-term complication after total hip arthroplasty [61]. It occurs with all types of materials and in almost all prosthetic systems. Revision total hip arthroplasty often presents surgeons with the difficult task of restoring bone loss at the site [62]. Therefore, the use of bone allograft in revision hip arthroplasty has gained acceptance [62–65]. Monitoring the incorporation and vitality of bone allograft is difficult by conventional imaging methods, however [66,67]. CT and MRI usually do not play a significant role in such clinical settings because of artifacts induced by the metal prosthesis. Similarly, conventional nuclear medicine modalities possess suboptimal spatial resolution in assessing the viability of small grafts. [18F]-fluoride PET is proven to be able to monitor the viability of osseous structures [68,69]. For this reason, dynamic fluoride PET has been used with great success for the evaluation of bone allograft viability and metabolism [70,71]. It has been shown that fluoride PET is a sensitive method for the evaluation of bone formation in allogenic bone grafts early after hip revision arthroplasty [70,71]. In addition, [15O]-water PET can be used in the evaluation of bone blood flow to the allograft in such a clinical setting [71].

Summary

PET is an important imaging modality for assessing the success of arthroplasty. The discrepancy in the results reported by different groups is mainly caused by the specific variation in the diagnostic criteria used by these investigators. As optimal standards for diagnosing periprosthetic infection are adopted by the imaging community, FDG-PET should play a crucial role in distinguishing aseptic loosening from periprosthetic infection. In addition, PET might be useful in the evaluation of bone graft after revision arthroplasty.

References

[1] Andrews HJ, Arden GP, Hart GM, et al. Deep infection after total hip replacement. J Bone Joint Surg Br 1981;63:53–7.

[2] Maderazo EG, Judson S, Pasternak H. Late infections of total joint prostheses. A review and recommendation for prevention. Clin Orthop 1988; 229:131–42.

[3] Brown SR, Davies WA, DeHeer DH, et al. Long-term survival of McKee-Farrar total hip prostheses. Clin Orthop 2002;402:157–63.

[4] Mahomed NN, Barrett JA, Katz JN, et al. Rates and outcomes of primary and revision total hip replacement in the United States Medicare population. J Bone Joint Surg Am 2003;85:27–32.

[5] Furnes O, Lie SA, Espehaug B, et al. Hip disease and the prognosis of total hip replacements. A review of 53,698 primary total hip replacements reported to the Norwegian Arthroplasty Register 1987–99. J Bone Joint Surg Br 2001;83:579–86.

[6] Fehring TK, Cohen B. Aspiration as a guide to sepsis in revision total hip arthroplasty. J Arthroplasty 1996;11:543–7.

[7] Spangehl MJ, Younger ASE, Masri BA, et al. Diagnosis of infection following total hip arthroplasty. J Bone Joint Surg Am 1997;79:1587–8.

[8] Barrack RL, Jennings RW, Wolfe MW, et al. The value of preoperative aspiration before total knee revision. Clin Orthop 1997;345:8–16.

[9] Kraemer WJ, Saplys R, Waddell JP, et al. Bone scan, gallium scan, and hip aspiration in the diagnosis of infected total hip arthroplasty. J Arthroplasty 1993;8:611–6.

[10] Reinartz P, Mumme T, Hermanns B, et al. Radionuclide imaging of the painful hip arthroplasty. J Bone Joint Surg Br 2005;87:465–70.

[11] Palestro CJ, Roumanas P, Swyer AJ, et al. Diagnosis of musculoskeletal infection using combined In-111 labeled leukocyte and Tc-99m SC marrow imaging. Clin Nucl Med 1992;17: 269–73.

[12] Mulamba LAH, Ferrant A, Lencers N, et al. Indium-111-leukocyte scanning in the evaluation of painful hip arthroplasty. Acta Orthop Scand 1983;54:695–7.

[13] Achong DM, Oates E. The computer-generated bone marrow subtraction image: a valuable adjunct to combined in-111 WBC/Tc-99m in sulfur colloid scintigraphy for musculoskeletal infection. Clin Nucl Med 1994;19:188–93.

[14] Palestro CJ, Kim CK, Swyer AJ, et al. Total-hip arthroplasty: periprosthetic indium-111 labeled leukocyte activity and complementary technetium-99m-sulfur colloid imaging in suspected infection. J Nucl Med 1990;31:1950–4.

[15] Alazraki NP. Diagnosing prosthetic joint infection. J Nucl Med 1990;31:1955–7.

[16] Bakheet SM, Saleem M, Powe J, et al. F-18 fluorodeoxyglucose chest uptake in lung inflammation and infection. Clin Nucl Med 2000;25: 273–8.

[17] Zhuang H, Cunnane ME, Ghesani NV, et al. Chest tube insertion as a potential source of false-positive FDG-positron emission tomographic results. Clin Nucl Med 2002;27:285–6.

[18] Dadparvar S, Anderson GS, Bhargava P, et al. Paraneoplastic encephalitis associated with cystic teratoma is detected by fluorodeoxyglucose positron emission tomography with negative magnetic resonance image findings. Clin Nucl Med 2003;28:893–6.

[19] Yu JQ, Kumar R, Xiu Y, et al. Diffuse FDG uptake in the lungs in aspiration pneumonia on positron emission tomographic imaging. Clin Nucl Med 2004;29:567–8.

[20] Bleeker-Rovers CP, de Kleijn E, Corstens FHM, et al. Clinical value of FDG PET in patients with fever of unknown origin and patients suspected of focal infection or inflammation. Eur J Nucl Med Mol Imaging 2004;31:29–37.

[21] Tsai YF, Wu CC, Su CT, et al. FDG PET CT features of an intraabdominal gossypiboma. Clin Nucl Med 2005;30:561–3.

[22] Nguyen QH, Szeto E, Mansberg R, et al. Paravertebral infection (phlegmon) demonstrated by FDG dual-head coincidence imaging in a patient with multiple malignancies. Clin Nucl Med 2005;30:241–3.

[23] Yu JQ, Kung JW, Potenta S, et al. Chronic cholecystitis detected by FDG-PET. Clin Nucl Med 2004;29:496–7.

[24] Zhuang H, Alavi A. 18-Fluorodeoxyglucose positron emission tomographic imaging in the detection and monitoring of infection and inflammation. Semin Nucl Med 2002;32:47–59.

[25] Zhuang H, Yu JQ, Alavi A. Applications of fluorodeoxyglucose-PET imaging in the detection of infection and inflammation and other benign disorders. Radiol Clin North Am 2005;43:121–34.

[26] De Winter F, Gemmel F, Van De Wiele C, et al. 18-Fluorine fluorodeoxyglucose positron emission tomography for the diagnosis of infection in the postoperative spine. Spine 2003;28:1314–9.

[27] Meller J, Koster G, Liersch T, et al. Chronic bacterial osteomyelitis: prospective comparison of F-18-FDG imaging with a dual-head coincidence camera and In-111-labelled autologous leucocyte scintigraphy. Eur J Nucl Med 2002;29: 53–60.

[28] Guhlmann A, Brecht-Krauss D, Suger G, et al. Fluorine-18-FDG PET and technetium-99m antigranulocyte antibody scintigraphy in chronic osteomyelitis. J Nucl Med 1998;39:2145–52.

[29] Kalicke T, Schmitz A, Risse JH, et al. Fluorine-18 fluorodeoxyglucose PET in infectious bone diseases: results of histologically confirmed cases. Eur J Nucl Med 2000;27:524–8.

[30] Temmerman OPP, Heyligers IC, Hoekstra OS, et al. Detection of osteomyelitis using (18)FDG and positron emission tomography. J Arthroplasty 2001;16:243–6.

[31] Zhuang H, Duarte PS, Pourdehand M, et al. Exclusion of chronic osteomyelitis with F-18

fluorodeoxyglucose positron emission tomographic imaging. Clin Nucl Med 2000;25:281–4.

[32] Gratz S, Dorner J, Fischer U, et al. F-18-FDG hybrid PET in patients with suspected spondylitis. Eur J Nucl Med Mol Imaging 2002;29:516–24.

[33] Keidar Z, Militianu D, Melamed E, et al. The diabetic foot: initial experience with F-18-FDG PET/CT. J Nucl Med 2005;46:444–9.

[34] Koort JK, Makinen TJ, Knuuti J, et al. Comparative F-18-FDG PET of experimental Staphylococcus aureus osteomyelitis and normal bone healing. J Nucl Med 2004;45:1406–11.

[35] Jones-Jackson L, Walker R, Purnell G, et al. Early detection of bone infection and differentiation from post-surgical inflammation using 2-deoxy-2-[(18)F]-fluoro-D-glucose positron emission tomography (FDG-PET) in an animal model. J Orthop Res 2005;23(6):1484–9.

[36] Sahlmann CO, Siefker U, Lehmann K, et al. Dual time point 2-F-18 fluoro-2′-deoxyglucose positron emission tomography in chronic bacterial osteomyelitis. Nucl Med Commun 2004; 25:819–23.

[37] Xiu Y, Yu JQ, Cheng E, et al. Sarcoidosis demonstrated by FDG PET imaging with negative findings on gallium scintigraphy. Clin Nucl Med 2005;30:193–5.

[38] Chacho TK, Zhuang H, Nakhoda KZ, et al. Application of fluorodeoxyglucose positron emission tomography in the diagnosis of infection. Nucl Med Commun 2003;24:615–24.

[39] Chacko TK, Zhuang HM, Alavi A. FDG-PET is an effective alternative to WBC imaging in diagnosing and excluding orthopedic infections [abstract]. J Nucl Med 2002;43:458.

[40] Schiesser M, Stumpe KDM, Trentz O, et al. Detection of metallic implant-associated infections with FDG PET in patients with trauma: correlation with microbiologic results. Radiology 2003; 226:391–8.

[41] Zhuang H, Duarte PS, Pourdehnad M, et al. The promising role of F-18-FDG PET in detecting infected lower limb prosthesis implants. J Nucl Med 2001;42:44–8.

[42] Reddy S, Hochhold J, Pill S, et al. The value of FDG-PET imaging in the evaluation of infection associated with hip arthroplasty. J Nucl Med 2005;46:324P.

[43] Vanquickenborne B, Maes A, Nuyts J, et al. The value of (18)FDG-PET for the detection of infected hip prosthesis. Eur J Nucl Med Mol Imaging 2003;30:705–15.

[44] Stumpe K, Nötzli H, Zanetti M, et al. FDG PET for differentiation of infection and aseptic loosening in total hip replacements: comparison with conventional radiography and three-phase bone scintigraphy. Radiology 2004;231:333–41.

[45] Zhuang H, Chacko TK, Hickeson M, et al. Persistent non-specific FDG uptake on PET imaging following hip arthroplasty. Eur J Nucl Med Mol Imaging 2002;29:1328–33.

[46] Revell PA, Weightman B, Freeman MA, et al. The production and biology of polyethylene wear debris. Arch Orthop Trauma Surg 1978;91: 167–81.

[47] Kisielinski K, Cremerius U, Reinartz P, et al. Fluorodeoxyglucose positron emission tomography detection of inflammatory reactions due to polyethylene wear in total hip arthroplasty. J Arthroplasty 2003;18:528–32.

[48] Kisielinski K, Reinartz P, Mumme T, et al. The FDG-PET demonstrates foreign body reactions to particulate polyethylene debris in uninfected knee prostheses. Nuklearmedizin 2004;43:N3–6.

[49] Chacko TK, Zhuang H, Stevenson K, et al. The importance of the location of fluorodeoxyglucose uptake in periprosthetic infection in painful hip prostheses. Nucl Med Commun 2002;23: 851–5.

[50] Mumme T, Reinartz P, Alfer J, et al. Diagnostic values of positron emission tomography versus triple-phase bone scan in hip arthroplasty loosening. Arch Orthop Trauma Surg 2005;125: 322–9.

[51] Chacko TK, Zhuang H, Nakhoda KZ, et al. Applications of fluorodeoxyglucose positron emission tomography in the diagnosis of infection. Nucl Med Commun 2003;24:615–24.

[52] De Winter F, Van de Wiele C, De Clercq D, et al. Aseptic loosening of a knee prosthesis as imaged on FDG positron emission tomography. Clin Nucl Med 2000;25:923.

[53] Van Acker F, Nuyts J, Maes A, et al. FDG-PET, 99mtc-HMPAO white blood cell SPET and bone scintigraphy in the evaluation of painful total knee arthroplasties. Eur J Nucl Med 2001;28: 1496–504.

[54] Heiba SI, Luo JQ, Sadek S, et al. Attenuation correction induced artifact in F-18 FDG PET imaging following total knee replacement. Clin Positron Imaging 2000;3:237–9.

[55] Manthey N, Reinhard P, Moog F, et al. The use of F-18 fluorodeoxyglucose positron emission tomography to differentiate between synovitis, loosening and infection of hip and knee prostheses. Nucl Med Commun 2002;23:645–53.

[56] Love C, Marwin SE, Tomas MB, et al. Diagnosing infection in the failed joint replacement: a comparison of coincidence detection F-18-FDG and In-111-labeled leukocyte/Tc-99m-sulfur colloid marrow imaging. J Nucl Med 2004;45:1864–71.

[57] Goerres GW, Schmid DT, Eyrich GK. Do hardware artefacts influence the performance of head and neck PET scans in patients with oral cavity squamous cell cancer? Dentomaxillofac Radiol 2003;32:365–71.

[58] Bockisch A, Beyer T, Antoch G, et al. Positron emission tomography/computed tomography-imaging protocols, artifacts, and pitfalls. Mol Imaging Biol 2004;6:188–99.

[59] Kamel EM, Burger C, Buck A, et al. Impact of metallic dental implants on CT-based attenuation correction in a combined PET/CT scanner. Eur Radiol 2003;13:724–8.

[60] Halpern BS, Dahlbom M, Waldherr C, et al. Cardiac pacemakers and central venous lines can induce focal artifacts on CT-corrected PET images. J Nucl Med 2004;45:290–3.

[61] Rubash HE, Sinha RK, Shanbhag AS, et al. Pathogenesis of bone loss after total hip arthroplasty. Orthop Clin North Am 1998;29:173–86.

[62] Gamradt SC, Lieberman JR. Bone graft for revision hip arthroplasty: biology and future applications. Clin Orthop 2003;417:183–94.

[63] Toms AD, Barker RL, Jones RS, et al. Impaction bone-grafting in revision joint replacement surgery. J Bone Joint Surg Am 2004;86:2050–60.

[64] Schreurs BW, Arts JJ, Verdonschot N, et al. Femoral component revision with use of impaction bone-grafting and a cemented polished stem. J Bone Joint Surg Am 2005;87:2499–507.

[65] Leopold SS, Jacobs JJ, Rosenberg AG. Cancellous allograft in revision total hip arthroplasty. A clinical review. Clin Orthop 2000;371:86–97.

[66] Heekin RD, Engh CA, Vinh T. Morselized allograft in acetabular reconstruction. A postmortem retrieval analysis. Clin Orthop 1995;319:184–90.

[67] Hooten Jr JP, Engh CA, Heekin RD, et al. Structural bulk allografts in acetabular reconstruction. Analysis of two grafts retrieved at postmortem. J Bone Joint Surg Br 1996;78:270–5.

[68] Schliephake H, Berding G, Knapp WH, et al. Monitoring of graft perfusion and osteoblast activity in revascularised fibula segments using [18F]-positron emission tomography. Int J Oral Maxillofac Surg 1999;28:349–55.

[69] Hawkins RA, Choi Y, Huang SC, et al. Evaluation of the skeletal kinetics of fluorine-18-fluoride ion with PET. J Nucl Med 1992;33:633–42.

[70] Piert M, Winter E, Becker GA, et al. Allogenic bone graft viability after hip revision arthroplasty assessed by dynamic [18F]fluoride ion positron emission tomography. Eur J Nucl Med 1999;26:615–24.

[71] Sorensen J, Ullmark G, Langstrom B, et al. Rapid bone and blood flow formation in impacted morselized allografts: positron emission tomography (PET) studies on allografts in 5 femoral component revisions of total hip arthroplasty. Acta Orthop Scand 2003;74:633–64.

POSITRON
EMISSION
TOMOGRAPHY

PET Clin 1 (2006) 107–121

Nonprosthesis Orthopedic Applications of ¹⁸F Fluoro-2-Deoxy-D-Glucose PET in the Detection of Osteomyelitis

Johannes Meller, MD[a],*, Carsten Oliver Sahlmann, MD[a],
Torsten Liersch, MD[b], Peter Hao Tang, BA[c], Abass Alavi, MD[c]

- Clinical background
  Bacterial osteomyelitis
- Pathophysiologic basis of
  [¹⁸F]2-fluoro-2-deoxy-D-glucose uptake in
  infection and inflammation
  Metabolic basis for
  [¹⁸F]2-fluoro-2-deoxy-D-glucose uptake
  Biodistribution
  Uptake of [¹⁸F]2-fluoro-2-deoxy-D-glucose
  in inflammatory cells
  Influence of serum glucose levels
  and insulin
  Summary
- Uptake of [¹⁸F]2-fluoro-2-deoxy-D-glucose
  during fracture healing and after
  bone surgery
  Physiology of bone healing
  Preclinical studies
  Clinical studies
- Clinical studies in osteomyelitis
  Acute osteomyelitis
  Chronic osteomyelitis
  Chronic recurrent multifocal osteomyelitis
- Summary
- References

Imaging for the diagnosis of orthopedic inflammation and infection dates back to the 1970s when modern imaging techniques were introduced. To this day, a three-phase bone scan is commonly used in the evaluation of OM of the intact bone. With the advent of white blood cell (WBC) labeling techniques, a relatively specific modality for orthopedic infection became available in the late 1970s.

The complexities of labeling WBCs, poor spatial resolution, and the difficulties in differentiating between soft tissue and bone involvement are major limitations of this method.

It has long been recognized that FDG accumulates not only in malignant tissues but at the sites of inflammation and infection, but systematic assessment of this method in diagnosing infection has

[a] Department of Nuclear Medicine, University of Göttingen, Robert Koch-Straße 40, D- 37075, Göttingen, Germany
[b] Department of General Surgery, University of Göttingen, Göttingen, Germany
[c] Division of Nuclear Medicine, Department of Radiology, Hospital of the University of Pennsylvania, 110 Donner Building, 3400 Spruce Street, Philadelphia, PA 19104, USA
* Corresponding author.
E-mail address: jmeller@med.uni-goettingen.de (J. Meller).

doi:10.1016/j.cpet.2006.01.004

only been undertaken over the past decade. This review describes the impact of FDG-PET in the diagnosis of non–prosthesis-related orthopedic infection as reported in the literature.

Clinical background

Bacterial osteomyelitis

OM is an acute or chronic inflammatory process of the bone marrow and adjacent bone attributable to pyogenic organisms. It is usually classified into several types based on the patient's age, onset of disease, route of infection, and etiology.

Known predisposing factors for OM are diabetes mellitus, AIDS, intravenous drug abuse, alcoholism, chronic steroid use, immunosuppression, chronic joint disease, any recent orthopedic surgery or open fractures, and the presence of prosthetic orthopedic devices [1,2].

Dependent on the route of inoculation and infections agents, OM is divided into hematogenous (endogenous) and nonhematogenous (exogenous) types. Hematogenous OM of an intact bone is seen most often in the extremities in neonates and children and in the spine of immunocompromised patients (spondylodiscitis). Nonhematogenous OM, which is appropriately better termed *ostitis* because the bone marrow is only infrequently involved, is the consequence of contiguous spread of infection from the adjacent soft tissue infection.

Bacterial types found in hematogenous OM include *Staphylococcus aureus*, *Streptococcus* variants, *Haemophilus influenzae*, and *Enterobacter* species. Exogenous OM (ostitis) is more often caused by *S aureus*, *Enterobacter* species, and *Pseudomonas* species [1–5].

Based on the appropriate clinical settings, the onset of symptoms, and the degree of inflammation, the process is described as acute, subacute, or chronic [1–4]. The distinction between acute OM and chronic osteomyelitis (COM) is somewhat arbitrary. Some patients with an acute clinical course show histologic findings suggestive of chronic disease, and during exacerbation of COM, focal polymorphonuclear infiltration would suggest acute infection [3].

Acute hematogenous osteomyelitis

Hematogenous OM is an infection caused by bacterial seeding from the blood. This occurs primarily in children and in the intact bone. The most common site of infection is the metaphysis of the long bones, which is highly vascular. The process begins with the implantation of microorganisms and a neutrophilic response. This is accompanied by local edema, vasospasm, and thrombosis. Segmental ischemic necrosis or sequestrum may follow soon after the process starts. The infection may be localized, or it may spread through the periosteum, cortex, marrow, and cancellous tissue. Depending on the child's age and the blood supply to the epiphysis, the process may or may not affect the adjacent joint. In children between the ages of 1 and approximately 16 years, the blood supply to the metaphysis and epiphysis is separate; therefore, spread of the microorganisms to the adjacent joint is rare. Conversely, in infants less than 1 year of age and in adults, there is a common blood supply to the metaphysis and epiphysis, and no growth plate barrier exists in this population. The presence of this communication facilitates the spread of infection to adjacent joints [1–6].

Acute exogenous osteomyelitis (ostitis)

The bone is highly resistant to infection, which can only occur as a result of direct contact between bone tissue and bacteria during trauma or surgery. Bacteria like *S aureus* adhere to the damaged bone by expressing various binding components, such as collagen, fibrinonectin, and others. Once the microorganisms adhere to the bone, they express phenotypic resistance to antimicrobial drugs, which may partly explain the high failure rate of antibiotic therapy of such infections [6].

Bone invasion by microorganisms is facilitated by focal osteolysis, which is caused by activated osteoclasts that are stimulated by cytokines released from the inflammatory cells. The disintegration of the surrounding bone matrix caused by proteolytic enzymes secreted by phagocytes further propagates bacterial invasion. Secondarily, the process may affect the bone marrow and lead to bone marrow phlegmon and other complications similar to those described for hematogenous OM. Clinical manifestations of ostitis are often localized compared with hematogenous OM, and multiple organisms are often noted at the site [1,2,4,5].

Chronic osteomyelitis

There is no generally accepted definition for COM, which is an expression that best describes bone and marrow infections and is based on histologic, clinical, and etiologic parameters [2,4,5]. COM is frequently the result of inadequate treatment of acute hematogenous OM or may follow exogenous bacterial contamination caused by trauma or surgical procedures. In contrast to acute OM, COM is predominantly characterized by the presence of lymphocytic and plasmacellular infiltrates and a variable amount of necrosis and osteosclerosis. In chronic recurrent cases, neutrophil infiltration may also be present. The presence of necrotic tissue may lead to draining fistulas or to organization in the medullary cavity, forming Brodie's abscesses [1,2,5]. Although, clinically, there is a frequent overlap between acute and chronic inflammatory changes, COM can be assumed if evidence of infection is present for more than 2 to 6 weeks. [1,3,5,7].

Vertebral osteomyelitis

Spondylodiscitis is an infection of the intervertebral disk and the adjacent vertebral bodies. The most commonly affected site is the lumbar spine. The disease occurs more frequently in older patients, especially in those who are immunocompromised. Most cases are caused by hematogenous bacterial spread from a distant site; however, in recent years, such infections have been noted after back surgery. The clinical course is usually rather subacute; therefore, the diagnosis is often delayed. The microorganisms are introduced by the arterial rather than the venous routes, and early infection is usually located in the subchondral zone of the end plate of the vertebral body, an area that is richly supplied with nutrient end arteries. The infection usually rapidly spreads to the adjacent vertebra above or below the disk space. Pyogenic spondylodiscitis virtually always involves two adjacent segments of the spine [3].

Chronic osteomyelitis and the diabetic foot

Approximately 15% of diabetics develop foot OM, which most commonly involves the metatarsal bones and proximal phalanges. In addition to impaired leukocyte function in these patients, OM is often the consequence of a condition called the "diabetic foot." Diabetic foot is a complex bone and joint disorder that involves the foot and ankle in patients with long-standing diabetes caused by neuropathy that affects the peripheral sensory, motor, and autonomic nerves. Eventually, this disorder leads to repetitive unnoticed damage and trauma without protective reflexes, imbalances in the arch of the foot with altered weight distribution and foot pressures, and deficient sweat production that causes thick and dry skin and callus formation in areas of pressure. Neuropathy combined with impaired arterial circulation and repetitive trauma is the major contributor to skin fissures and ulcer formation. More than 90% of OM of the foot in diabetics occurs as a result of infected ulcers, which lead to subsequent COM of the adjacent bone [6].

Pathophysiologic basis of [^{18}F]2-fluoro-2-deoxy-D-glucose uptake in infection and inflammation

Metabolic basis for [^{18}F]2-fluoro-2-deoxy-D-glucose uptake

FDG is structurally an analogue of glucose; therefore, it is taken up according to the degree of glycogen in the body.

The uptake of glucose and FDG into mammalian cells takes place via three mechanisms of transport. The first, passive diffusion, is of minor importance for human tissues. The second, active transport by a Na^+-dependent glucose transporter, is of importance in the kidney epithelial cells and intestinal tract. The third and most significant pathway for FDG to enter human cells is active transport mediated by facilitated glucose transporters (GLUT-1–10) [8].

Once FDG has entered the cell, it is subsequently phosphorylated to 2'-FDG-6 phosphate by the hexokinase enzyme. In contrast to glucose-6-phosphate, 2'-FDG-6 phosphate is not a substrate for the enzymes of the glycolytic pathway or the pentose-phosphate shunt. In tissues with low concentrations of the glucose-6-phosphatase enzyme, such as the heart and brain, the uptake of 2'-FDG-6 phosphate increases over time. In other organs with high concentrations of the enzyme, such as the liver, the uptake of 2'-FDG-6 phosphate decreases after the rapid initial accumulation [9,10].

Biodistribution

FDG is filtrated in the glomeruli in the kidneys, and only a small fraction is reabsorbed by the renal tubular cells. Rapid clearance of the tracer from the vascular compartment results in a high target-to-background ratio within a short time; therefore, imaging can start as early as 30 to 60 minutes after injection.

A high accumulation of FDG is always seen in the brain, especially in the gray matter. Cardiac uptake is unpredictable in patients who have fasted before dose administration. If the patient exercises before the administration of the tracer, muscular uptake may be high. Because of renal excretion, the kidney, pelvis, and urinary bladder are usually visualized on FDG scans. Variable levels of FDG uptake are seen in the gastrointestinal tract, which may interfere with correct interpretation of the scan, is likely attributable to smooth muscle peristalsis, and can be reduced by the administration of N-butylscopolamine [11].

Tracer uptake in the reticuloendothelial system (RES), and especially in the red bone marrow, is significant. In patients with fever, bone marrow uptake is usually high, probably as a consequence

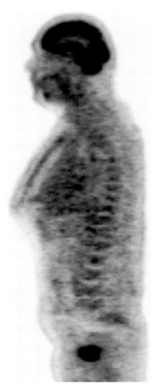

Fig. 1. In patients with normal hematopoietic activity, there is usually a low degree of uptake in the axial bone marrow. If the bone marrow is activated by cytokines, as in this patient with fever of unknown origin, the uptake may be high, which may result in false-negative findings. In this patient with OM, FDG uptake in the lesions was obscured because of increased background activity within the third and fourth vertebral bodies of the lumbar spine (PET sagittal view).

of interleukin-dependent upregulation of glucose transporters [Fig. 1] [12]. The cortical bone and cavity of the long tubular bones are usually free of activity [Fig. 2]. Systematic studies on the uptake in the normal synovia of healthy individuals have not been reported in literature. It has been recognized, however that a faint FDG uptake is almost always present in the synovial portion of the joints. The uptake may be related to normal glucose consumption in the tissue, but osteoarthritis should be considered as the basis for this observation [13].

Uptake of [¹⁸F]2-fluoro-2-deoxy-D-glucose in inflammatory cells

It has long been recognized that FDG accumulates not only in malignant tissues but at the sites of inflammation and infection [14,15]. A few studies have made an attempt to clarify the mechanism of FDG uptake in the inflammatory cells in vitro [16–18]. In these experiments, mixed preparations

of WBCs or pure preparations of neutrophils and mononuclear cells were used for this purpose. In these research studies, the labeling efficiency ranged from 40% to 80% [16–18]. If a mixed population of nonstimulated WBCs is incubated with FDG, labeling is predominantly attributable to granulocytic uptake, accounting for 78% to 87% of the activity in the preparation. The labeling efficiency depends on the amount of activity in the media and the experimental temperature, with the maximum labeling efficiency achievable at 37°C. The uptake increases within the first 60 minutes [16, 18]. The extent of uptake by neutrophilic granulocytes is inversely proportional to the glucose concentration in the labeling medium [16]. Insulin, even in high concentrations, does not increase the uptake in the inflammatory cells [17].

If neutrophilic granulocytes are stimulated by substances like phorbol myristate or the chemotactic peptide N-formyl-methionyl-leucyl-phenylalanine (f-MLP) for a relatively short period of 60 minutes, a significant increase in FDG uptake is noted compared with nonstimulated cells [16,18].

The labeling of WBCs with FDG is not stable, and an elution of 27% to 35% within the first 60 minutes has been reported [16,18]. Osman and Danpure [16] demonstrated that after the initial intracellular uptake and phosphorylation of FDG in WBCs, it is then dephosphorylated by the

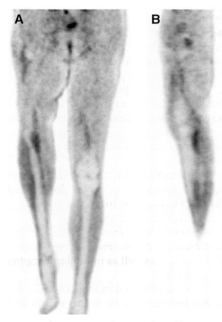

Fig. 2. Normal pattern in the peripheral bone on FDG-PET. The long bones are usually free of any activity. The uptake near the cortical bone in the maximal projection image (*A*) is clearly related to vascular activity, as demonstrated on the sagittal view (*B*).

glucose-6-phosphatase and leaves the cells again. Because of this poor stability, cells labeled with FDG in vitro are not suited for clinical application, although some authors have advocated their use for clinical purposes [17]. The functionality of the labeled cells after reinjection is another open question.

Currently, autoradiographic data about differential uptake of FDG in inflammatory cell elements are limited. In a microautoradiographic study, Kubota and colleagues [19] demonstrated that the tracer uptake in tumors was partly attributable to newly formed granulation tissue and activated macrophages associated with tumor necrosis and growth. In this study, the FDG uptake of nonneoplastic cell elements was even higher than the accumulation of the tracer in viable tumor cells. In another report, FDG uptake in postmigratory and activated leukocytes in lobar pneumonia was autoradiographically shown to be localized within neutrophils [20].

Activated lymphocytes in concanavalin A–mediated acute inflammatory tissues showed increased uptake of FDG in in vitro and in vivo models [21]. In an animal model of bacterial infection induced by inoculation with *Escherichia coli*, autoradiographs showed that the highest [^{3}H]-FDG uptake was in the area of inflammatory cell infiltration surrounding the necrotic region [22].

In recent years, many aspects of the molecular basis of FDG uptake in WBCs have been successfully clarified. As already discussed, the transport of glucose and structurally related substances like FDG into mammalian cells is mediated by facultative glucose transporters (GLUT-1–10) [8]. GLUT-1 is the most common isotype and is thought to play a major role in the basal glucose supply of many fetal and adult tissues. The expression of GLUT-1 has been especially demonstrated in the brain, the cells of the blood-brain barrier, and the blood, particularly in erythrocytes but also in the leukocyte fraction [23].

GLUT-1 seems to be the target of many cytokines and the most important isotype for our understanding of FDG uptake in WBCs, especially after stimulation. Overexpression of GLUT-1 after stimulation with cytokines or mutagens has already been demonstrated in vitro in murine and human macrophages [24–26] as well as in human lymphocytes and neutrophils [27,28].

GLUT-1 is located predominantly in the plasma membrane but can also be found within intracellular vesicles [26]. After stimulation, the intracellular GLUT-1 pool can be translocated to the cell membrane, thus increasing glucose transport capacity within a relatively short time [12]. If human lymphocytes are stimulated with mitogens, this ef-

fect takes place as early as 30 minutes after the beginning of stimulation [29]. This may explain the early increase of FDG uptake in cultured WBCs in vitro.

In addition to these early stimulatory effects, the late (>24 hours) increase in FDG uptake in stimulated inflammatory cells in vitro is attributable to a gene-dependent de novo synthesis of GLUT-1. This has already been demonstrated on an mRNA and protein level for lymphocytes [27], where the maximal overexpression of GLUT-1 was observed for murine and human monocytes as late as 48 hours after stimulation [24–26]. Similar results were found in neutrophilic granulocytes and cellular elements of granulation tissue, such as fibroblasts and the endothelium [30–33].

In human tuberculosis lesions, the GLUT-1–positive staining was often localized in the membranes of neutrophils and macrophages around necrotizing granulomas as well as in the cytoplasm. These cells also showed positive staining for the hexokinase II (HK-II) isoform, which is known to play a dominant role in the accelerated phosphorylation of FDG in tumor cells [28].

GLUT-3 has a high affinity for glucose and can be found in a wide range of tissues, especially in the kidney, the placenta, and the neurons in the brain, where it ensures a constant glucose supply even at low extracellular glucose concentrations [17].

In a monocyte-macrophage cell line, GLUT-3 affinity for glucose was found to be enhanced during the respiratory burst [34], whereas nonstimulated WBCs usually did not express this type of transporter [27].

Mochizuki and coworkers [35] used a suspension of *S aureus* in rats to induce soft tissue infection. Other animals were inoculated with allogenic hepatoma cells into the left calf muscle. The expression of glucose transporters (GLUT-1–5) was investigated by immunostaining the infectious and tumor tissues. In this study, the [^{14}C]FDG uptake was significantly higher in the tumor than in the inflammatory lesion. The tumor and inflammatory tissues highly expressed GLUT-1 and GLUT-3. The GLUT-1 expression level was, however, significantly higher in the tumor tissue than in the inflammatory tissue. The GLUT-3 levels tended to be higher in the inflammatory lesions than in the tumor, but the difference did not reach statistical significance.

Influence of serum glucose levels and insulin

High serum glucose levels decrease glucose uptake in experimental inflammatory and infectious lesions because of decreased GLUT-1 (inflammatory lesions of noninfectious origin) and GLUT-3 (inflammatory lesions of infectious origin) expression [36]. Whether or not this observation is of clinical

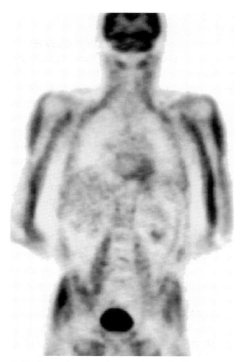

Fig. 3. FDG-PET images (coronal view) of a 72-year-old patient with spondylodiscitis in the lumbar spine. A false-negative result in this affected site is attributable to hyperinsulinemia. Maximal FDG uptake is found in the skeletal muscles by upregulation of the GLUT-4 isotype.

importance remains an open question. Based on their in vitro and in vivo data, Zhuang and coworkers [37] concluded that contrary to observations in malignant disorders, below a level of 250 mg/dL, elevated glucose concentration does not have a negative effect on FDG uptake in inflammatory cells.

Hyperinsulinemia increases the level of glucose uptake in GLUT-4–rich organs like the heart, fat, and muscles by translocation of GLUT-4 from intracellular vesicles to the membrane and therefore shifts the uptake from inflammatory lesions toward these tissues [36]. This mechanism leads to false-negative results in FDG-PET imaging [Fig. 3].

Summary

In summary, migratory and postmigratory inflammatory cells stimulated by cytokines show an overexpression of GLUT-1 and GLUT-3 and an activation of the glycolytic pathway. These mechanisms of enhanced FDG uptake are of essential importance in PET imaging of acute and chronic bacterial infection. Although the expression of glucose transporters is insulin sensitive to a certain degree, in vivo data indicate that serum glucose

levels below a certain level may not adversely affect the image quality for inflammatory lesions.

Uptake of [^{18}F]2-fluoro-2-deoxy-D-glucose during fracture healing and after bone surgery

Physiology of bone healing

Fracture healing is a complex process that involves the coordinated participation of several cell types. It begins with an inflammatory phase, followed by repair and remodeling, and culminates in the ability of bone to regain its original tissue structure. Fracture healing begins immediately after injury when interleukins and growth factors are released into the fracture hematoma by platelets and inflammatory cells. Growth factors are regulators of cellular proliferation, differentiation, and extracellular matrix synthesis during fracture repair. The most important of these are the bone morphogenetic proteins (BMPs), transforming growth factor-β (TGFβ), platelet-derived growth factor (PDGF), fibroblast growth factor (FGF), insulin-like growth factor (IGF), vascular endothelial growth factor (VEGF), and epidermal growth factor (EGF). Altered growth factor expression may be responsible for abnormal or delayed fracture repair. Intramembranous ossification occurs under the periosteum within a few days after an injury. Endochondral ossification occurs adjacent to the fracture site and spans a period of up to 1 month [38].

Preclinical studies

Systematic preclinical studies on FDG uptake in the healing bone after fracture and surgery are infrequently reported in the literature.

Jones-Jackson and coworkers [39] used a rabbit OM model and a dual–time-point FDG-PET protocol to differentiate between postsurgical inflammation and infection of the bone. Comparisons were made between noninfected and infected rabbits in which infection with *S aureus* was initiated at the time of surgery. Increased uptake of FDG was evident in the bone of all rabbits on day 1 after surgery; however, the standardized uptake value (SUV) could not be used to distinguish between the infected and uninfected groups until day 15.

Koort and colleagues [40] compared the natural course of bone healing after creating a metaphyseal defect in the tibia of rabbits without (control group) and after the inoculation of *S aureus* (OM group). Before surgery, the SUVs of FDG did not differ markedly between the right and left tibias. In the controls, uncomplicated bone healing was associated with a temporary increase in FDG uptake in the third week, with almost complete normalization by week 6. In the OM group, localized infection resulted in an intense continuous uptake of FDG, which was significantly higher than that of the healing and intact bones at weeks 3 and 6.

Clinical studies

The first clinical data on FDG uptake in the traumatized bone are concordant with those of the experimental observations [41–50]. Fig. 4 shows a false-positive finding in a patient with a history of fracture less than 3 weeks old [see Fig. 4].

In a series of 29 patients with known fractures, no false-positive findings were noted in 5 patients who underwent bone surgery within 3 to 28 weeks before FDG-PET with a coincidence camera [44].

In a study by Zhuang and coworkers [48] in 22 patients with fractures, 2 with a recent osteotomy showed false-positive FDG uptake, whereas a negative scan ruled out infection in the remaining 20 subjects.

In another report in 60 patients with suspected OM, FDG-PET allowed correct identification of OM in 25 patients, but 2 of 3 patients with false-positive findings had undergone bone surgery less than 6 weeks and 4 months before PET imaging [42].

In a prospective series of 16 patients with suspected spondylitis who underwent FDG-PET with a coincidence camera, one false-positive finding was

noted and was attributed to a vertebral fracture of unknown age [47].

In another prospective FDG-PET study of 57 patients with a history of previous spinal surgery, false-positive findings occurred in 2 of 27 patients without metallic implants within the first 6 months after surgery. A negative PET scan had a negative predictive value of 100% [43].

In a retrospective study in 37 patients with known fractures, the pattern and time course of abnormal FDG uptake after traumatic or surgical fracture were assessed. Fourteen patients had fractures or surgery within 3 months before FDG-PET, whereas 23 had fractures or surgical intervention more than 3 months before FDG-PET. FDG-PET showed normal uptake at the known fracture or surgical site(s) in 30 patients. In the 23 patients with fractures more than 3 months old, all but 1 showed no abnormally increased uptake. This patient had a complicated case of OM. Six of the 14 patients with a history of fracture less than 3 months old had abnormally increased FDG uptake despite normal fracture healing [49].

Schmitz and colleagues [50] evaluated FDG-PET findings in patients with osteoporosis and acute (<3 weeks) vertebral compression fractures. The results of blind scoring of FDG uptake at the fracture sites were compared with those of MRI, which served as the "gold standard." In 13 of 17 patients, MRI demonstrated an osteoporotic fracture. Twelve of 13 PET scans in these patients were scored as 0 or 1 (no uptake or uptake slightly increased) and were categorized as true-negative findings in patients with uncomplicated fractures. The maximum SUV ranged from 1.1 to 2.4. In the remaining 4 patients, MRI revealed a pathologic fracture caused by spondylodiscitis in 3 patients and by plasmocytoma in 1 patient. In these patients, FDG-PET scans were highly positive and the maximum SUV values ranged from 3.8 to 9.8.

In summary, less than 50% of patients with uncomplicated traumatic or surgical fractures demonstrate pathologic FDG uptake within the first 3 months after bone injury. During this time, interval reparative changes of the bone are usually characterized by low FDG uptake and by maximum SUV values less than 2. Intense uptake and higher maximum SUV values at a fracture site for longer than 3 months are suspicious for infection or other pathologic processes, such as malignancy. Our present knowledge about possible differences in the time course of enhanced FDG uptake after trauma to the bone in different sites is limited. The glucose metabolism of the axial and peripheral skeleton after trauma may be different. Another open question is how different mechanical forces at different sites may affect glucose metabolism of the healing

A

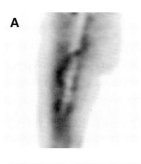

B

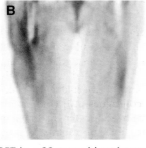

Fig. 4. FDG-PET in a 38-year-old patient with a recent fracture of the right femur and soft tissue infection of the surrounding soft tissue (*A*, sagittal view; *B*, coronal view). Although soft tissue infection was proven by surgery, the uptake in the bone was posttraumatic and not related to infection.

bone. In a study on postoperative fever, we noted distinct FDG uptake after an uncomplicated sternotomy in 3 patients up to 5 weeks after surgery, which could have been easily confused with the presence of OM [45].

Clinical studies in osteomyelitis

Acute osteomyelitis

Acute OM, especially that of the intact bone, can readily be diagnosed by the combination of physical examination, laboratory findings, and three-phase bone scanning or MRI. The role of FDG-PET in acute infection of the bone is limited, because conventional imaging techniques have a diagnostic accuracy of more than 90% [15,46].

In a study describing 15 patients with histopathologically proven OM, 7 had acute infection of the spine or the perpendicular skeleton. All cases in this highly selected patient population were detected by FDG-PET [51]. Except for these seven cases, publications about FDG-PET in acute OM have been limited to the animal models already described [39,40]. Without data of larger prospective studies, it is impossible to define a possible role for FDG-PET in the diagnosis of acute bone and marrow infection.

Chronic osteomyelitis

Using conventional imaging methods, including MRI and labeled leukocyte scanning, the diagnosis of COM remains a diagnostic challenge.

In the context of COM, bone scintigraphy is sensitive, and a negative bone scan can rule out infection in almost all cases. Conversely, a low specificity of 18% to 62% has been reported for the bone scan in the diagnosis of COM [46,52,53]. In vitro radiolabeled leukocytes or immunoscintigraphy with in vivo labeling antigranulocyte antibodies has proven to be accurate in the diagnosis of COM in the peripheral skeleton but lacks sensitivity and specificity in the axial bones [6,15].

The sites of chronic infection in the axial skeleton are usually characterized by an area of decreased activity on the WBC scan. This pattern is nondiagnostic for active inflammation because it may also be found in other conditions, such as healing OM, fibrosis, fatty bone marrow degeneration, metastases, primary tumors of the bone, and osteonecrosis [6,46]. Decreased uptake of labeled cells in infection of the axial skeletal compartment is poorly understood. This is likely attributable to relatively high uptake of FDG in the red marrow compared with the site of infection. Other explanations include microthrombotic occlusion and inflammatory compression of the blood capillaries,

which prevent the migration of labeled cells or antibodies to the site of infection [6,15,46]. Conversely, FDG uptake in active OM is usually enhanced, whereas glycolysis in the surrounding bone marrow is relatively low, which allows for the detection of lesions that are missed in WBC imaging [Figs. 5 and 6].

MRI has been recognized as an extremely sensitive modality for the detection of COM; compared with nuclear medicine techniques, it provides more accurate anatomic information about the extent of the process and possible complications [52,53]. The criteria used to identify inflammatory changes, such as the edema pattern on T2-weighted sequences and contrast enhancement after intravenous administration of gadolinium, are unspecific, however, and may produce false-positive results, especially in the first year after surgery. Furthermore, artifacts produced by metallic implants hinder correct interpretation [52,53].

Guhlmann and coworkers [54] were the first to publish a prospective study about the possible role of FDG-PET in the diagnosis of COM. They evaluated the results of FDG-PET and antigranulocyte antibody scintigraphy in 51 patients. COM was suspected if OM was recurrent or if symptoms lasted for more than 6 weeks. Patients who had undergone bone surgery within the past 2 years were excluded. In 31 patients, histologic findings

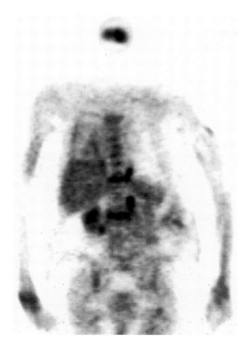

Fig. 5. FDG-PET images (coronal view) of a 62-year-old patient with multifocal OM of the spine and soft tissue involvement of the adjacent areas.

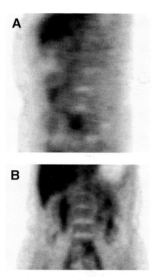

Fig. 6. FDG-PET images of a 48-year-old patient with OM of the ventral lumbosacral junction extending to the soft tissue. (*A*, sagittal view; *B*, coronal view).

or the results of bacterial culture were available. For image interpretation, a visual score was used. The findings were evaluated by two independent readers who were blinded to the final diagnosis. Excellent accuracy and interobserver agreement for both techniques (97% and 95% for FDG-PET and 86% and 92% for antigranulocyte antibody scintigraphy, respectively) were noted in the peripheral skeleton (n = 36). In the axial skeleton (n = 15), accuracy was significantly higher for FDG-PET (93% and 100%) than for antigranulocyte antibody scintigraphy (73% and 80%; $P < .05$).

In another publication by the same group, in 31 patients suspected of having COM in the peripheral (n = 21) or axial (n = 10) skeleton and having available histology results, the overall sensitivity and specificity of FDG-PET were 100% and 92%, respectively. The one false-positive case was in a patient with a soft tissue infection of the mandible. This was explained by a lack of the missing landmarks of FDG-PET in this region [55]. Again, patients with previous bone surgery within the past 12 months before PET imaging were excluded, which may explain the low rate of false-positive findings in this and the previous study.

Zhuang and colleagues [48] investigated 22 patients with possible COM (axial skeleton [n = 11] or peripheral skeleton [n=11]). The final diagnosis was made by surgical exploration or clinical follow-up during a 1-year period. FDG-PET correctly diagnosed all 6 patients with COM. There were two false-positive findings, resulting in a sensitivity, specificity, and accuracy of 100%, 87.5%, and 91%, re-

spectively. The two false-positive findings were caused by a recent osteotomy.

Kälicke and coworkers [51] reported the results of FDG-PET in 15 histologically confirmed cases of infection (8 with COM and 7 with acute OM). The authors provided no definition of acute and OM. The PET findings were evaluated by two independent readers, blinded to the results of other imaging modalities. Image interpretation was performed by using a semiquantitative score. FDG-PET yielded true-positive results in all 15 patients. The absence of negative findings in this series may raise questions concerning selection criteria, however.

De Winter and coworkers [41] prospectively evaluated the role of the dual-headed coincidence (DHC) imaging system versus the role of a dedicated PET device in 24 patients with suspected chronic orthopedic infection. A final diagnosis in this study was obtained by microbiologic proof in 11 patients and clinical follow-up in 13 patients. The sensitivity and specificity in this series were 100% and 86% for the dedicated PET and 89% and 96% for the DHC, respectively. These results indicate that DHC imaging, despite a lower imaging quality, can be used successfully in the evaluation of orthopedic infections in most cases.

The same group published a prospective study of 60 patients in whom COM, spondylodiscitis, or infection of a total joint prosthesis was suspected [42]. Microbiologic and histopathologic findings were available for 42 patients. In 24 patients, detailed clinical follow-up confirmed the diagnosis. Suspected COM was defined as a possible recurrence of previously known disease or the presence of typical symptoms for more than 6 weeks. Patients with recent bone surgery were not excluded. FDG images were evaluated visually by two independent readers blinded to the final diagnosis. Twenty-five patients had infection, and 35 did not. All 25 infections were correctly identified by both readers. There were four false-positive findings; in two of these cases, surgery had been performed less than 6 months before the study. The sensitivity and specificity for the 33 patients with a suspected infection of the axial skeleton were 100% and 90%, respectively. The sensitivity and specificity for the 13 patients with a suspected infection of the peripheral skeleton were 100% and 86%, respectively.

Schmitz and colleagues [56] performed FDG-PET in 16 patients with suspected spondylodiscitis. Surgery and histopathologic examination were performed in all patients. The FDG-PET findings were semiquantitatively graded and evaluated by two independent readers. Of the 16 patients, 12 had histopathologically confirmed spondylodiscitis. There were true-positive FDG-PET findings in all 12 of

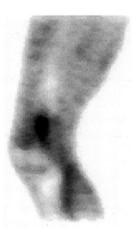

Fig. 7. FDG coincidence imaging with a DHC imaging system (sagittal slices) 30 minutes after injection of FDG (sagittal slices) in a 44-year-old patient with COM in the distal femur.

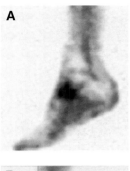
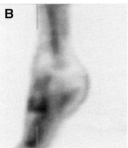

these patients. In the 4 patients without spondylodiscitis, FDG-PET showed three true-negative results and one false-positive result.

Meller and coworkers [44] published a prospective analysis of 29 consecutive nondiabetic patients who were studied for possible COM and underwent combined indium (In)-111 WBC imaging and FDG-PET with a DHC imaging system. In 4 patients, bone surgery had been performed within the past 6 months. All patients complained of localized symptoms for more than 6 weeks. Image interpretation was performed semiquantitatively by two investigators who were blinded to the results of other diagnostic modalities and the final diagnosis. Of 34 regions with suspected infection, 13 were localized in the axial skeleton and 21 in the peripheral skeleton [Figs. 7 and 8]. COM was proven in 10 of 34 regions and subsequently excluded in 24 of 34 regions. The final diagnosis was established by histologic examination and culture in 18 regions and by MRI and clinical follow-up in 16 regions. The sensitivity of PET imaging was 100%, and the specificity was 95%. Results of

Fig. 9. FDG-PET (dual-time protocol 30 minutes and 60 minutes after injection, sagittal slices) in a 63-year-old patient with tarsal COM. The extent of the inflammatory uptake and the SUV decreased with time (*A*, 30 minutes after injection, maximum SUV = 4.22; *B*, 90 minutes after injection, maximum SUV = 3.58).

[111]In WBC imaging were inferior, especially in the axial skeleton.

In a prospective study of 17 patients with histopathologically proven COM of the axial skeleton, our group used a dual-time protocol to evaluate the tracer kinetics of FDG in chronic bacterial OM compared with the kinetics of bone metastases [Figs. 9–11]. In all infectious lesions, increased FDG uptake was seen at 30 and 90 minutes after the injection of FDG. In COM lesions, the maximum SUV and mean SUV between 30 and 90 minutes after injection remained stable or decreased in 16 of 17 patients. Changes in the maximum SUV and mean SUV between 30 and 90 minutes were

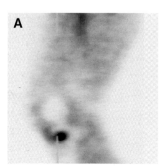
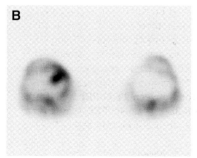

Fig. 8. FDG coincidence imaging with a DHC imaging system (sagittal slices) 120 minutes after injection of FDG in a 35-year-old patient with COM in the right proximal tibia (*A*, sagittal view; *B*, transversal view).

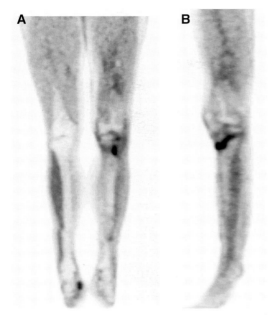

Fig. 10. FDG-PET images of a 67-year-old patient with COM in the proximal tibia 90 minutes after injection of FDG (*A*, coronal view; *B*, sagittal view). Note the presence of osteoarthritis of the right hallux.

highly significant (*P*<.05). In 1 patient, the maximum SUV and mean SUV increased over the time. The histologic examination of this patient revealed multiple foreign body granulomas in addition to a mononuclear infiltrate. In malignant lesions, the maximum SUV and mean SUV between 30 and 90 minutes after injection increased. From these limited results, we concluded that a dual-time protocol should allow differentiation between infectious and malignant lesions of the spine in most cases [57].

The great potential of FDG-PET in postoperative patients can be derived from the data provided by de Winter and colleagues [43] in 57 consecutive patients with a history of previous spinal surgery who underwent FDG-PET in the postoperative period. Of these patients, 15 had a spinal infection, whereas infection could be ruled out in the others. Images were semiquantitatively and visually scored by two blinded independent readers. Using the most sensitive cutoff values, sensitivity, specificity, and accuracy were 100%, 81%, and 86%, respectively, for visual and semiquantitative scoring.

Direct comparisons between FDG-PET and MRI are of great importance, because PET may overcome some of the limitations of MRI as described previously.

One patient who developed COM and ostitis after repeated osteosynthesis in a fibular transplant underwent MRI, antigranulocyte antibody scintig-

raphy, and FDG PET. Infection of the fibular transplant was demonstrated by PET but not by the other methods [58].

Our group prospectively studied 12 patients with suspected COM. FDG-PET was as sensitive as but more specific than MRI (100% versus 60%) [44]. In a retrospective study of 14 patients after surgery of the spine, the sensitivity of FDG-PET and MRI was 87%, whereas the specificity of PET was superior to that of MRI (100% versus 85%) [59]. Larger prospective studies in a population of patients that should include cases after bone surgery are therefore clearly warranted.

Chronic recurrent multifocal osteomyelitis

Chronic recurrent multifocal osteomyelitis (CRMO) has been described as a self-limited relapsing inflammatory condition histologically characterized by a mononuclear cell infiltrate and usually affecting children and adolescents [6]. A nonbacterial origin for CRMO is probable but not proven. Most of the lesions are seen in the long bones, especially in the tibia. The clavicle is often bilaterally involved. Fig. 12 shows one of the three patients who underwent combined bone scintigraphy, antigranulocyte antibody scintigraphy, and FDG-PET in our institution. Although the bone scan was positive in all known lesions, the antigranulocyte antibody scintigraphy showed decreased up-

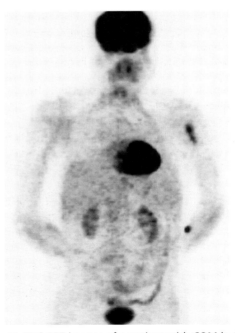

Fig. 11. FDG-PET images of a patient with COM in the proximal left humerus 90 minutes after injection of FDG (coronal view).

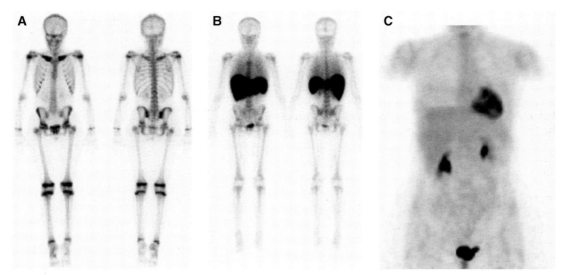

Fig. 12. CRMO in both clavicles in an 18-year-old male patient. The bone scan (*A*) was positive in the clavicular lesions, and the antigranulocyte antibody scintigraphy (*B*) showed decreased uptake at the sites of inflammation. (*C*) Maximal projection FDG-PET image was completely negative.

take at the sites of inflammation. FDG-PET was completely negative in all lesions, indicating low metabolic activation of the lymphoplasmacellular infiltrate [see Fig. 12].

Summary

FDG-PET imaging seems to have excellent sensitivity in the detection of COM. A normal scan virtually rules out infection. FDG-PET is superior to scintigraphy with labeled blood cells in the diagnosis of COM in the axial skeleton and should thus be considered the method of choice for this indication. This seems to hold true for peripheral lesions as well, but the number of cases published to date is too small to permit a final conclusion. FDG-PET is likely to become the standard technique in the diagnosis of COM in the near future.

Compared with labeled blood cells, FDG-PET has some important advantages:

- Diagnosis can be performed within a short period (1–2 hours after injection).
- From a theoretic point of view, it can be assumed that labeled WBCs only accumulate in COM if sufficient blood flow is present at the site of infection and if the chemotactic-guided emigration of labeled cells from the blood pool to the inflammatory tissue is still ongoing. FDG, as a small molecule, is expected to be much more independent of microcirculatory changes and can label activated postmigratory granulocytes and mononuclear cells in the inflammatory tissue sites.

- Compared with conventional gamma camera imaging, PET offers higher spatial and contrast resolutions. As a rule, no FDG uptake can be observed in the normal bone and uptake in the axial bone marrow is low. The target-to-background ratio in infectious lesions on the FDG scan is thus higher than that of the labeled images.
- When labeled cells are used to delineate infectious processes in the axial skeleton, the diseased sites appear to be negative compared with the surrounding background because of uptake of WBCs in the hematopoietic bone marrow. This pattern results in low sensitivity for the labeled cell technique. Conversely, active OM in the axial skeleton can be clearly visualized by FDG-PET in almost all cases because of substantially increased glucose metabolism at the sites of infection compared with the normal bone marrow.
- Uptake of labeled WBCs in the hematopoietic bone marrow in the peripheral skeleton poses a problem when using labeled leukocytes. Low-grade infection in these areas may be missed because of unfavorable target-to-background ratios with this technique. FDG shows minimal uptake in the bone marrow of the peripheral skeleton; therefore, such confusion can be avoided.
- Low-grade infection or infection with purely mononuclear or granulomatous infiltrates may be missed on WBC scanning. It is well known that FDG uptake is generally preserved in these conditions and is independent of chemotactic stimuli.

Traumatic or surgical fracture has been found to be the most frequent cause of false-positive findings on FDG-PET in the context of evaluation for COM. Careful interpretation of the scan using semiquantitative or quantitative methods may avoid false-positive results in many cases, but differentiating between infection and inflammation is an issue that may not be feasible with PET, especially in the first 4 to 6 weeks after trauma.

Early data indicate that FDG-PET may be more specific than MRI in diagnosing COM. In general, MRI can only show tissue edema and hyperperfusion and is thus not specific in this context. FDG-PET is taken up in postmigratory inflammatory cells, and the uptake in the tissue is independent of such phenomena. This allows a unique opportunity to detect the primarily elements at the site of infection. Larger prospective studies are clearly warranted to clarify this matter.

The significance of low-uptake lesions on FDG-PET with a normal appearance on MRI has not been fully elucidated, because these are usually categorized as false-positive findings and may not require further investigation. It may well be possible that lesions with low FDG uptake represent ongoing infection and are related to exacerbation of a latent disease.

The use of PET-CT in the assessment of infections processes should further enhance the role of the technique for this indication. In particular, this methodology should be of great importance in separating soft tissue infection from that of the musculoskeletal structures.

References

[1] Lew DP, Waldvogel FA. Osteomyelitis. N Engl J Med 1997;336(14):999–1007.

[2] Lew DP, Waldvogel FA. Osteomyelitis. Lancet 2004;364(9431):369–79.

[3] Waldvogel FA, Medoff G, Swartz MN. Osteomyelitis: a review of clinical features, therapeutic considerations and unusual aspects. N Engl J Med 1970;282(4):316–22.

[4] Waldvogel FA, Vasey H. Osteomyelitis: the past decade. N Engl J Med 1980;303(7):360–71.

[5] Mader JT, Shirtliff M, Calhoun JH. Staging and staging application in osteomyelitis. Clin Infect Dis 1997;25(6):1303–9.

[6] Becker W. Imaging osteomyelitis and the diabetic foot. Q J Nucl Med 1999;43(1):9–20.

[7] Schauwecker DS. The scintigraphic diagnosis of osteomyelitis. AJR Am J Roentgenol 1992;158(1):9–18.

[8] Shepherd PR, Kahn BB. Glucose transporters and insulin action: implications for insulin resistance and diabetes mellitus. N Engl J Med 1999;341(4):248–57.

[9] Sokoloff L, Reivich M, Kennedy C, et al. The (14C) deoxyglucose method for the measurement of local cerebral glucose utilisation: theory, procedure and normal values in the conscious and anesthetized albino rat. J Neurochem 1977;28(6):897–916.

[10] Pauwels EK, Sturm EJ, Bombardieri E, et al. Positron-emission tomography with fluorodeoxyglucose. Part I. Biochemical uptake mechanism and its implication for clinical studies. J Cancer Res Clin Oncol 2000;126(10):549–59.

[11] Stahl A, Weber WA, Avril N, et al. Effect of N-butylscopolamine on intestinal uptake of fluorine-18-fluorodeoxyglucose in PET imaging of the abdomen. Nuklearmedizin 2000;39(8):241–5.

[12] Baldwin SA, Kan O, Whetton AD, et al. Regulation of the glucose transporter GUT1 in mammalian cells. Biochem Soc Trans 1994;22(3):814–7.

[13] von Schulthess GK, Stumpe KDM, Engel-Bicik I. Clinical PET imaging of inflammatory diseases. In: von Schulthess GK, editor. Clinical positron emission tomography (PET). Philadelphia: Lippincott Williams & Wilkins; 2000. p. 229–48.

[14] Tahara T, Ichiya Y, Kuwabara Y, et al. High-fluorodeoxyglucose uptake in abdominal abscesses: a PET study. J Comput Assist Tomogr 1989;13(5):829–31.

[15] Becker W, Meller J. The role of nuclear medicine in infection and inflammation. Lancet Infect Dis 2001;1(1):326–33.

[16] Osman S, Danpure HJ. The use of 2-fluoro-2-deoxy-D-glucose as a potential in vitro agent for labelling human granulocytes for clinical studies by positron emission tomography. Int J Radiat Appl Instrum 1992;19(2 Pt B):183–90.

[17] Forstrom LA, Mullan BP, Hung JC, et al. ^{18}F-FDG labelling of human leucocytes. Nucl Med Commun 2000;21(7):691–4.

[18] Lehmann K, Meller J, Behe M, et al. F-18-FDG uptake in granulozyten: basis der F-18-FDG szintigraphie. Nuklearmedizin 2001;40(3):V168 [in German].

[19] Kubota R, Yamada S, Kubota K, et al. Intratumoral distribution of fluorine-18-fluorodeoxyglucose in vivo: high accumulation in macrophages and granulocytes studied by microautoradiography. J Nucl Med 1992;33(7):1972–80.

[20] Jones HA, Sriskandan S, Peters AM, et al. Dissociation of neutrophil emigration and metabolic activity in lobar pneumonia and bronchiectasis. Eur Respir J 1997;10(4):795–803.

[21] Ishimori T, Saga T, Mamede M, et al. Increased (18)F-FDG uptake in a model of inflammation: concanavalin A-mediated lymphocyte activation. J Nucl Med 2002;43(5):658–63.

[22] Sugawara Y, Gutowski TD, Fisher SJ, et al. Uptake of positron emission tomography tracers in experimental bacterial infections: a comparative biodistribution study of radiolabeled FDG, thy-

midine, L-methionine, 67Ga-citrate, and 125I-HSA. Eur J Nucl Med 1999;26(4):333–41.

[23] Gould GW, Holman GD. The glucose transporter family: structure, function and tissue-specific expression. Biochem J 1993;295:329–41.

[24] Gamelli RL, Liu H, He LK, et al. Augmentations of glucose uptake and glucose transporter-1 in macrophages following thermal injury and sepsis in mice. J Leukoc Biol 1996;59(5):639–47.

[25] Fukuzumi M, Shinomiya H, Shimizu Y, et al. Endotoxin-induced enhancement of glucose influx into murine peritoneal macrophages via GLUT1. Infect Immun 1996;64(1):108–12.

[26] Malide D, Davies-Hill TM, Levine M, et al. Distinct localisation of GLUT-1 and -5 in human monocyte-derived macrophages: effects of cell activation. Am J Physiol 1998;274(3 Pt 1):E516–26.

[27] Chakrabarti R, Jung CY, Lee TP, et al. Changes in glucose transport and transporter isoforms during the activation of human peripheral blood lymphocytes by phytohemagglutinin. J Immunol 1994;152(6):2660–8.

[28] Mamede M, Higashi T, Kitaichi M, et al. FDG uptake and PCNA, Glut-1, and Hexokinase-II expressions in cancers and inflammatory lesions of the lung. Neoplasia 2005;7(4):369–79.

[29] Jacobs DB, Lee TP, Jung CY, et al. Mechanism of mitogen-induced stimulation of glucose transport in human peripheral blood mononuclear cells. J Clin Invest 1989;83(2):437–43.

[30] Pekala P, Marlow M, Heuvelman D, et al. Regulation of hexose transport in aortic endothelial cells by vascular permeability factor and tumor necrosis factor-alpha, but not by insulin. J Biol Chem 1990;265(30):18051–4.

[31] Cornelius P, Marlowe M, Pekala PH. Regulation of glucose transport by tumor necrosis factor-α in cultured murine 3T3–L1 fibroblasts. J Trauma 1990;30(12 Suppl):S15–20.

[32] Tan AS, Ahmed N, Berridge MV. Acute regulation of glucose transport after activation of human peripheral blood neutrophils by phorbol myristate acetate, fMLP, and granulocyte-macrophage colony-stimulating factor. Blood 1998;91(2):649–55.

[33] Bird TA, Davies A, Baldwin SA, et al. Interleukin 1 stimulates hexose transport in fibroblasts by increasing the expression of glucose transporters. J Biol Chem 1990;265(23):13578–83.

[34] Ahmed N, Kansara M, Berridge MV. Acute regulation of glucose transport in a monocyte-macrophage cell line: Glut-3 affinity for glucose is enhanced during the respiratory burst. Biochem J 1997;327:369–75.

[35] Mochizuki T, Tsukamoto E, Kuge Y, et al. FDG uptake and glucose transporter subtype expressions in experimental tumor and inflammation models. J Nucl Med 2001;42(10):1551–5.

[36] Zhao S, Kuge Y, Tsukamoto E, et al. Fluorodeoxyglucose uptake and glucose transporter expression in experimental inflammatory lesions and malignant tumours: effects of insulin and glucose loading. Nucl Med Commun 2002;23(6):545–50.

[37] Zhuang HM, Cortes-Blanco A, Pourdehnad M, et al. Do high glucose levels have differential effect on FDG uptake in inflammatory and malignant disorders? Nucl Med Commun 2001;22(10):1123–8.

[38] Einhorn TA. The cell and molecular biology of fracture healing. Clin Orthop 1998;355(Suppl):S7–21.

[39] Jones-Jackson L, Walker R, Purnell G, et al. Early detection of bone infection and differentiation from post-surgical inflammation using 2-deoxy-2-[(18)F]-fluoro-d-glucose positron emission tomography (FDG PET) in an animal model. J Orthop Res 2005;23(6):1484–9.

[40] Koort JK, Makinen TJ, Knuuti J, et al. Comparative 18F-FDG PET of experimental Staphylococcus aureus osteomyelitis and normal bone healing. J Nucl Med 2004;45(8):1406–11.

[41] de Winter F, Van de Wiele C, Vandenberghe S, et al. Coincidence camera FDG imaging for the diagnosis of chronic orthopedic infections: a feasibility study. J Comput Assist Tomogr 2001;25(2):184–9.

[42] de Winter F, van de Wiele C, Vogelaers D, et al. Fluorine-18 fluorodeoxyglucose-position emission tomography: a highly accurate imaging modality for the diagnosis of chronic musculoskeletal infections. J Bone Joint Surg Am 2001;83(5):651–60.

[43] de Winter F, Gemme F, Van De Wiele C, et al. 18-Fluorine fluorodeoxyglucose positron emission tomography for the diagnosis of infection in the postoperative spine. Spine 2003;28(12):1314–9.

[44] Meller J, Köster G, Liersch T, et al. Chronic bacterial osteomyelitis—prospective comparison of 18 FDG-imaging with a double head coincidence camera (DHCC) and In-111 labeled autologous leucocytes. Eur J Nucl Med 2002;29(1):53–60.

[45] Meller J, Sahlmann CO, Lehmann K, et al. F-18-FDG hybrid camera PET in patients with postoperative fever. Nuklearmedizin 2001;41(1):22–9.

[46] Meller J, Siefker U, Becker W. Nuklearmedizinische Diagnostik erregerbedingter Skeletterkrankungen [Scientific diagnosis of bacterial skeletal diseases]. Nuklearmedizin 2002;25(2):122–32 [in German].

[47] Gratz S, Dörner J, Fischer U, et al. 18F-FDG hybrid PET in patients with suspected spondylitis. Eur J Nucl Med 2002;29(4):516–24.

[48] Zhuang H, Duarte PS, Pourdehand M, et al. Exclusion of chronic osteomyelitis with F-18 fluorodeoxyglucose positron emission tomographic imaging. Clin Nucl Med 2000;25(4):281–4.

[49] Zhuang H, Sam JW, Chacko TK, et al. Rapid normalization of osseous FDG uptake following traumatic or surgical fractures. Eur J Nucl Med Mol Imaging 2003;30(8):1096–103.

[50] Schmitz A, Risse JH, Textor J, et al. FDG PET findings of vertebral compression fractures in osteoporosis: preliminary results. Osteoporos Int 2002;13(9):755–61.

[51] Kälicke T, Schmitz A, Risse JH, et al. Fluorine-18 fluorodeoxyglucose PET in infectious bone diseases: results of histologically confirmed cases. Eur J Nucl Med 2000;27(5):524–8.

[52] Kaim A, Ledermann HP, Bongartz G, et al. Chronic post-traumatic osteomyelitis of the lower extremity: comparison of magnetic resonance imaging and combined bone scintigraphy/immunoscintigraphy with radiolabelled monoclonal antigranulocyte antibodies. Skeletal Radiol 2000;29(7):378–86.

[53] Kaim AH, Gross T, von Schulthess GK. Imaging of chronic posttraumatic osteomyelitis. Eur Radiol 2003;13(7):1750–2.

[54] Guhlmann A, Brecht Krauss D, Suger G, et al. Fluorine-18-FDG PET and technetium-99m antigranulocyte antibody scintigraphy in chronic osteomyelitis. J Nucl Med 1998;39(12):2145–52.

[55] Guhlmann A, Brecht-Krauss D, Suger G, et al. Chronic osteomyelitis: detection with FDG PET and correlation with histopathologic findings. Radiology 1998;206(3):749–54.

[56] Schmitz A, Risse JH, Grunwald F, et al. Fluorine-18 fluorodeoxyglucose positron emission tomography findings in spondylodiscitis: preliminary results. Eur Spine J 2001;10(6):534–9.

[57] Sahlmann CO, Siefker U, Lehmann K, et al. Dual time point 2-[^{18}F]fluoro-2'-deoxyglucose ([^{18}F]FDG)-PET in chronic bacterial osteomyelitis (COM). Nucl Med Commun 2004;25(8):819–23.

[58] Robiller FC, Stumpe KD, Kossmann T, et al. Chronic osteomyelitis of the femur: value of PET imaging. Eur Radiol 2000;10(5):855–8.

[59] Siefker U, Sahlmann CO, Lehmann K, et al. F-18-FDG PET im Vergleich zur MRT bei der Primärdiagnostik und postoperativen Kontrolle bei chronischer bakterieller Osteomyelitis (COM). Nuklearmedizin 2004;43(3):V116 [in German].

ELSEVIER
SAUNDERS

POSITRON
EMISSION
TOMOGRAPHY

PET Clin 1 (2006) 123–130

Application of 18F-Fluorodeoxyglucose and PET in Evaluation of the Diabetic Foot

John Hochhold, MD[a,b], Hua Yang, MD[a,b],
Hongming Zhuang, MD, PhD[a,b,c], Abass Alavi, MD[a,b,*]

- Epidemiology and pathophysiology of
  diabetic foot
  Plain film
  Conventional scintigraphy
  Radiolabeled white cell imaging

  MRI
  18F-fluorodeoxyglucose PET
- Summary
- References

Osteomyelitis is one of the major complications of a neuropathic diabetic foot. Despite long-term antibiotic therapy and surgical interventions, osteomyelitis often remains refractory and leads to a chronic infection in most diabetic patients with this disorder. In general, diabetic foot progresses from neuropathy to Charcot's disease and is commonly associated with skin ulcers. Eventually, these patients present with findings that are suggestive of acute osteomyelitis or chronic osteomyelitis, which may lead to wet or dry gangrene. Clinical symptoms and signs of deep-seated foot infection, in contrast to nonneuropathic conditions, are often atypical or absent, which may obscure the diagnosis. In particular, underlying neurodegenerative osteoarthropathy can often mislead clinicians and further delay a timely diagnosis. Obviously, accurate and timely differentiation of osseous infections from those of the soft tissues alters clinical management in this setting. Early diagnosis and expeditious intense treatment of osteomyelitis may prevent amputation, which is the most feared complication in these patients. Because of the complex anatomic structure of the midfoot, where the abnormalities caused by Charcot's disease are often noted, postsurgical inflammatory changes and frequent soft tissue infections make the diagnosis quite difficult. 18F-fluorodeoxyglucose (FDG) PET has been used successfully to diagnose osteomyelitis at various sites in nondiabetic patients. Its utility in assessing complications of the diabetic foot, as documented in the literature, is the subject of this report.

This work is partially supported by National Institutes of Health grant 5R01DK063579-04 (A. Alavi).
a Division of Nuclear Medicine, Department of Radiology, University of Pennsylvania School of Medicine, Philadelphia, PA 19104, USA
b Hospital of the University of Pennsylvania, 110 Donner Building, 3400 Spruce Street, Philadelphia, PA 19104, USA
c The Children's Hospital of Philadelphia, Philadelphia, PA 19104, USA
* Corresponding author. Division of Nuclear Medicine, Hospital of the University of Pennsylvania, 110 Donner Building, 3400 Spruce Street, Philadelphia, PA 19104.
E-mail address: abass.alav@uphs.upenn.edu (A. Alavi).

doi:10.1016/j.cpet.2006.03.001

Epidemiology and pathophysiology of diabetic foot

The prevalence of foot ulcers in diabetics is estimated at between 5% and 10%, with approximately 15% of this population developing osteomyelitis at some point [1]. The total annual cost of diabetic peripheral neuropathy and its complications in the United States is estimated to be between $4.6 and $13.7 billion [2]. Up to 27% of the direct medical cost of diabetes may be attributed to diabetic peripheral neuropathy [2].

The timely recognition and subsequent management of osteomyelitis can reduce morbidity from complications, which include amputation and the dissemination of infection [3]. Bone resection and partial amputations may still be necessary, but early diagnosis, followed by aggressive antibiotic therapy and minor surgical procedures, can prevent above-ankle amputation and reduce the length of hospitalization [4].

Bone infection in the diabetic foot occurs by the local spread of microorganisms from an overlying ulcer [5]. Deep space infections are generally suspected in patients with a persistent superficial ulcer, systemic signs of toxicity, inflammation far from the skin wound, and persistently elevated inflammatory markers despite appropriate therapy [5]. Systemic signs of toxicity, such as fever and chills, may be absent in up to two thirds of patients with osteomyelitis among patients with diabetes, however [6]. Up to 50% of diabetic patients with a deep foot infection do not have an elevated white cell count [7–9]. Published data suggest that an erythrocyte sediment rate greater than 70 is specific but not sensitive for osteomyelitis [8,10,11]. Palpation of bone through an ulcer is also specific for the diagnosis of osteomyelitis but is insensitive for detecting this disorder [12].

Adding further complexity to the diagnosis of osteomyelitis is the fact that acute neurodegenerative osteoarthropathy, also known as Charcot joint, can present with signs, symptoms, and findings similar to those of infections [10]. There are currently two theories proposed to describe the pathophysiology of Charcot joint. According to the neurotraumatic theory, neuropathy leads to diminished proprioception which, in combination with repetitive trauma, results in bone and joint destruction. In the neurovascular theory, it is postulated that an autonomically mediated vascular reflex results in hyperemia and periarticular osteopenia. Altered weight bearing follows and leads to microfracture, ligamentous laxity, and, finally, bony destruction [13].

The importance of diagnosing osteomyelitis early in its course and initiating potentially limb-saving treatment cannot be overemphasized in diabetic patients. Therefore, a noninvasive imaging technique that accurately provides the diagnosis can play an important role in this setting.

Plain film

Conventional radiography is an inexpensive modality that is used in the workup of suspected pedal osteomyelitis. The classic signs of osteomyelitis on radiographs include periosteal thickening, bony sequestra, and involucra [14]. Infection can fester for 10 to 14 days before signs become evident on plain films [14,15], however, and 30% to 50% of the bone must be destroyed before osteomyelitis can be diagnosed radiographically [16]. The sensitivity of plain film to diagnose osteomyelitis in patients with foot ulcers ranges from 28% to 93%, and the specificity ranges from 25% to 92% [16]. Acute neurodegenerative osteoarthropathy may demonstrate relatively few signs on plain film [17]. As the process becomes chronic, a constellation of findings, including local osteoporosis, subchondral cysts, erosions, diastasis, and subluxation, becomes evident [13]. In the late stage of neurodegenerative osteoarthropathy, sclerosis and bony fusion are seen [16].

Obviously, the overall low sensitivity and delay in making the radiographic diagnosis of osteomyelitis can result in suboptimal management of these patients.

Conventional scintigraphy

Three-phase bone scintigraphy using technetium (Tc)-99m-methyl diphosphonate (MDP) as a radiotracer demonstrates a sensitivity that ranges from 69% to 100% for detecting osteomyelitis in the diabetic foot, which make it an excellent and widely available screening test [3,11,18–20]. A normal three-phase bone scan almost certainly excludes the possibility of osteomyelitis [19]. Increased radiotracer uptake on the blood flow and blood volume and enhanced uptake on the delayed phase of this study are suggestive of underlying osteomyelitis. Bone scintigraphy has a low specificity, however [3,11,18–22]. In addition, enhanced radiotracer activity on all three phases of this procedure can be seen in a variety of other osseous diseases, including fracture and the acute phase of Charcot foot [23].

Some authors suggest using a fourth-phase bone scan, for which images of the feet are acquired approximately 24 hours after radiotracer injection [24,25]. The finding of radiotracer uptake that is persistent or more intense on 24-hour images than that on the 3-hour scans is suggestive of osteomyelitis and increases the overall accuracy of bone scanning for osteomyelitis, from 80% to 85% in one series [24]. This pattern has been ascribed to the relative predominance of woven over lamellar bone in osteomyelitis [26].

Bone scintigraphy is a sensitive but nonspecific technique in the evaluation of pedal osteomyelitis in patients with diabetes. The addition of a fourth phase may increase overall accuracy and specificity at the expense of sensitivity. Delayed imaging (24 hours) is more time-consuming and is inconvenient to patients with a diabetic foot because of the necessity of making an additional visit a day later.

Radiolabeled white cell imaging

Radiolabeled white cell scintigraphy has been used for the evaluation of a suspected infectious process. The white cell preparation is incubated with either of two radiotracer compounds: Tc-99m–hexamethylpropyleneamine oxime (HMPAO) or indium-111-oxine. When labeled with Tc-99m, images are generally acquired 3 to 4 hours after injection, and when using indium-111–labeled white blood cells, images are taken 24 hours after administration of these cells [27].

Several series have compared the diagnostic accuracy of tagged white cell images with those of the three-phase bone scans [3,11,18,22]. The sensitivities of white cell imaging in these series are comparable to bone scintigraphy, with values ranging from 79% to 100%. The specificity of white cell imaging ranges from 29% to 78% and is generally greater than that of bone scintigraphy for excluding osteomyelitis in the diabetic foot [3,11,18,20, 22,27]. Increased radiolabeled leukocyte uptake has been described in fracture, areas of marrow hyperplasia, and neurodegenerative osteoarthropathy, however [3,11,18,22,28]. Delineating areas of increased bone marrow activity with a sulfur colloid scan before leukocyte imaging can increase the sensitivity and specificity for detecting pedal osteomyelitis [28,29]. Despite the advantages of leukocyte scintigraphy, precise localization of the sites of infection is difficult because of poor spatial resolution of the technique, especially when distinguishing between cellulitis and osteomyelitis is of clinical concern [18,22]. Tc-99m-HMPAO–labeled white blood cells may theoretically provide superior anatomic localization; therefore, higher sensitivity and specificity can be achieved with this modality compared with the indium-111–labeled leukocyte scans [27]. The disadvantages of this technique include the high cost, time required to prepare the labeled cells and then to perform the test, and danger of contamination with microorganisms and reinjection of human blood products [26].

MRI

Over the past 2 decades, MRI has been an effective modality for the evaluation of osteomyelitis in the feet of diabetic patients, with sensitivity values that range from 77% to 100% [30–33]. Areas of bone marrow edema, as defined by decreased signal on T1-weighted images and increased signal on T2-weighted images, suggest the diagnosis of osteomyelitis. Osseous enhancement after the intravenous administration of gadolinium has been evaluated and is of minimal benefit in characterizing osteomyelitis [30,34,35]. Despite these advances, bone marrow edema attributable to osteomyelitis can also be seen with a variety of pathologic processes, such as fracture, postsurgical repair, and acute neurodegenerative osteoarthropathy. As a result, the specificity varies between 40% and 100% [19,23,35,36]. To improve the specificity of the technique, several authors have advocated the addition of some other criteria, such as the presence of a cutaneous ulcer underlying the region of bone marrow edema, sinus tract, and cortical interruption [35,37,38]. It has been suggested that the anatomic location of the bone marrow edema has diagnostic significance. Bone infections more commonly occur at the first distal phalanx, first and fifth metatarsals, and calcaneus [39]. Bone marrow edema in the midfoot is viewed as suggestive of Charcot joint, because infection infrequently involves this anatomic site [39]. Focal marrow signal abnormalities in the midfoot adjacent to a site of soft tissue infection that is different from other areas of presumed neuropathic disease may be considered representative of an infectious process [35].

MRI has a significant advantage over other techniques for providing excellent spatial resolution and precise anatomic localization of the abnormal sites. The specificity of MRI varies substantially and may depend on the experience of the interpreting physician, the set of diagnostic criteria being used, and the strength of the magnet. A subset of patients with metal implants, such as orthopedic hardware, cannot undergo MRI and should be assessed with other techniques.

18F-fluorodeoxyglucose PET

In recent years, the role of FDG-PET has been increasingly examined for detecting and localizing sites of infection throughout the human body [38,40–47]. PET possesses a number of advantages over other scintigraphic techniques. It has the ability to acquire and display tomographic images within a reasonably short time. PET allows for improved anatomic localization and coregistration with CT and MRI scans. The overall duration of the procedure from the administration of FDG to the generation of tomographic images is substantially shorter than that of conventional bone or leukocyte scintigraphy. The presence of metallic implants, such as a pacemaker, orthopedic prosthesis, or medical port, does not adversely affect the quality of the images provided by PET. The preparation of the final product is relatively simple; therefore, the risk of contamination with microorganisms is almost nonexistent with modern techniques. Finally, the cost is substantially less than that of white blood cell imaging.

The most commonly used PET radiotracer is FDG, which serves as a marker of intracellular metabolism and has been shown to be taken up by the inflammatory cells. Therefore, FDG has been shown to accumulate intensely at the sites of acute and chronic osteomyelitis with a high degree of consistency [48–52].

Diabetic patients with Charcot foot deformities have been evaluated by FDG-PET with promising results. In an investigation involving 39 Charcot foot lesions confirmed by surgery, 37 were accurately identified by a dedicated full-ring PET camera with a sensitivity of 95%. In contrast, a coincidence PET camera detected 30 of the 39 lesions with a sensitivity of 77%, whereas MRI revealed 31 of these lesions with a sensitivity of 79% [53]. Importantly, the authors noted that PET can provide accurate results in patients with metal implants, who are precluded from undergoing MRI. In addition, the authors believe that PET can accurately distinguish osteomyelitis and Charcot neuroarthropathy [53].

Keidar and colleagues [52] reported their preliminary experience with FDG-PET/CT scans of the feet of diabetic patients. A total of 18 sites in 14 subjects were evaluated in this study. The diagnosis of osteomyelitis was confirmed by histo-

pathologic studies or a combination of clinical and radiographic follow-up. PET correctly detected osteomyelitis in 8 of 8 sites and soft tissue infection in 5 of 5 sites. The standard uptake values (SUVs) of areas of osteomyelitis ranged from 1.7 to 13 and from 1.7 to 11.1 in soft tissue infections [52]. In the same study, the authors noted that CT revealed osteomyelitis in 7 of 8 sites and soft tissue infection in 4 of 5 sites, which was less accurate than the PET findings. Therefore, FDG-PET/CT allowed accurate diagnosis of all sites of infection [52].

Preliminary data from our institution also suggest that FDG-PET is an accurate imaging modality in the evaluation of osteomyelitis in the diabetic foot [54]. A total of 39 subjects with diabetes were recruited for this ongoing study. Based on these data, FDG-PET has successfully demonstrated osteomyelitis in 9 of 10 subjects and correctly excluded osteomyelitis in 22 of 24 subjects. The sensitivity and specificity of PET are therefore 90% and 91.7%, respectively [54]. Our data demonstrated that FDG-PET can clearly distinguish osteomyelitis from soft tissue infection [Figs. 1 and 2].

Most patients with diabetes in spite of optimal control of the disease are noted to have hyperglycemia before FDG is administered. In such circumstances, the question arises as to whether elevated serum glucose levels at the time of this test could affect FDG uptake at the sites of infection and inflammation. Published data from our center suggest that the quality of FDG-PET scans as well as the degree of uptake with serum glucose levels up to 250 mg/dL may not be affected when this test is used to detect infection. In fact, there may be a possible negative association between serum glucose levels and the degree of FDG uptake in malignant lesions and a positive relation in inflam-

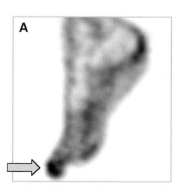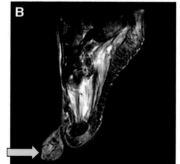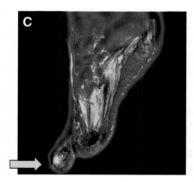

Fig. 1. A 39-year-old woman with a history of diabetes underwent an FDG-PET scan to evaluate for possible osteomyelitis. The sagittal PET scan (*A*) shows a focus of hypermetabolism in the distal hallux of the right foot, suggesting active osteomyelitis. The focally increased FDG activity corresponds well to the location of abnormal signal on MRI (*B*), which is further demonstrated by the PET/MRI fusion scan (*C*). The presence of osteomyelitis was subsequently confirmed by surgery, pathologic examination, and culture.

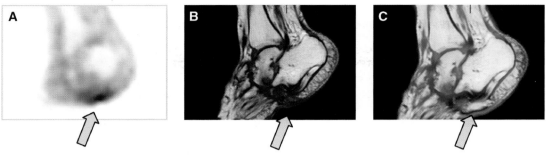

Fig. 2. A 47-year-old diabetic woman with a known pedal ulcer and suspicion for osteomyelitis. The FDG-PET scan (*A*) revealed superficially increased activity in the region of the ulcer without any abnormal activity in the bones. This activity corresponds to the abnormal signal in a region anterior to the calcaneus on MRI (*B*) and PET/MRI fusion (*C*). The bone biopsy and clinical follow-up results proved that this patient did not have osteomyelitis.

matory processes [55]. Consistent with these findings, animal experiments have demonstrated that high accuracy of FDG-PET in the diagnosis of osteomyelitis can be maintained without fasting in these models [56]. This is contrast to what has been observed with FDG-PET in the assessment of patients with cancer, where fasting is essential for generating high-quality images for diagnostic purpose. In the study of the diabetic foot by Keidar and colleagues [52], accurate interpretation was achieved in spite of glucose levels exceeding 200 mg/dL at the time of the PET scan in half of these patients. In fact, there were no false-negative results attributable to hyperglycemia in the population examined. Similarly, there was minimal difference in the PET results in the evaluation of Charcot lesions between those patients with normal levels and those with elevated serum sugar levels [53].

FDG-PET is more specific than a bone scan in the evaluation of osteomyelitis. Unlike bone scintigraphy, which shows significantly increased tracer uptake many months to years after traumatic fracture, no FDG activity is seen at these sites after 2 to 3 months [17]. Laboratory data in rabbits suggest that uncomplicated bone healing may demonstrate increased FDG uptake for up to 6 weeks after injury before returning to normal, whereas osteomyelitis is likely to demonstrate continuously rising SUVs [56]. Neurodegenerative osteoarthropathy poses a more serious challenge than fracture when infection is suspected, considering that moderately elevated FDG uptake has been demonstrated in Charcot joints [52,53,57]. FDG uptake in neurodegenerative osteoarthropathy tends to be diffuse, however, and generally involves the tarsal-metatarsal regions [58]. In addition, our initial analysis suggests that, on average, SUVs in the inflammatory regions of the Charcot foot seem to be lower than those in areas of infection. Our results are consis-

tent with those of the previous report by Hopfner and coworkers [53].

Quantification of radiotracer activity using maximum SUVs may potentially help to differentiate areas of infection from those of inflammation. More research is required to define clearly the role of quantitation techniques in differentiating infection from inflammation on the basis of threshold value. Also, no report has yet addressed the effects of walking, sitting, or lying flat after the administration of radiotracer and before imaging with PET.

New PET tracers that are designed to be specifically taken up at the sites of infection are currently being evaluated [59,60]. FDG has been labeled to leukocytes and shown to accumulate at the sites of inflammation and infection. Although this technique could theoretically have a higher sensitivity than conventional indium-111– or Tc-99m–labeled leukocyte scintigraphy because of the superior spatial resolution provided by PET compared with that of single photon emission computed tomography (SPECT), it suffers from the same logistic challenges described previously. In addition, the patterns of FDG-labeled cell uptake may not differ substantially from those of FDG in spite of the complexity of the procedure [61]. F-18–labeled ciprofloxacin has been studied in patients with culture-proven lower extremity bacterial infection [60]. Although the areas of infection demonstrated increased tracer concentration, the washout half-time was similar to that of noninfected tissue, which suggests that the degree of vascularity, as opposed to specific tracer binding to bacteria at the sites, is the basis for such accumulation. Although the concept is attractive, the clinical role of radiolabeled antibiotics is questionable at this time.

Gallium-68, a positron-emitting tracer, has been shown to accumulate at the site of bone healing at nearly the same intensity as normal bone; however, it accumulates to a greater extent in osteomyelitis [58,62]. Gallium-68 may thus be of value in clinical scenarios in which there is known bone healing but infection is also a concern.

Although FDG, and possibly 18F-labeled white cells, have the potential to image infection directly, hypoxia agents, such EF5 [2-(2-nitro-1[*H*]-imidazol-1-yl)-*N*-(2,2,3,3,3-pentafluoropropyl)-acetamide], are novel tracers that may provide indirect evidence of severe, anaerobic infection, particularly in the diabetic foot. EF5 undergoes hypoxia-dependent metabolism that results in the formation of cellular covalent drug adducts [63]. As such, it is considered a marker of hypoxia, and current clinical applications have focused on its role in delineating regions of tumor hypoxia [63–70]. Potential applications of EF5-PET in the diabetic foot include the diagnosis of anaerobic infection and monitoring the response to hyperbaric oxygen therapy in wound healing.

Summary

In spite of advances in modern imaging techniques, diagnosis of infection in the diabetic foot remains a major diagnostic challenge. FDG is increasingly being used as a noninvasive diagnosis modality for managing a variety of infectious processes and has demonstrated its unique role in detecting osteomyelitis in the diabetic foot compared with other conventional diagnostic tools. FDG-PET, combined with CT, has great promise for distinguishing osteomyelitis from other pathologic entities in the diabetic foot. Novel PET tracers also may further enhance the role of this modality for diagnosing infection and should provide an optimal understanding of the underlying pathologic mechanisms and help to develop effective treatment for these serious disorders.

References

[1] Boulton AJ, Vileikyte L. The diabetic foot: the scope of the problem. J Fam Pract 2000;49(Suppl):S3–8.

[2] Gordois A, Scuffham P, Shearer A, et al. The health care costs of diabetic peripheral neuropathy in the US. Diabetes Care 2003;26:1790–5.

[3] Levine SE, Neagle CE, Esterhai JL, et al. Magnetic resonance imaging for the diagnosis of osteomyelitis in the diabetic patient with a foot ulcer. Foot Ankle Int 1994;15:151–6.

[4] Lipsky BA. A current approach to diabetic foot infections. Curr Infect Dis Rep 1999;1:253–60.

[5] Lipsky BA. A report from the International Consensus on diagnosing and treating the infected diabetic foot. Diabetes Metab Res Rev 2004;20(Suppl 1):S68–77.

[6] Schinabeck MK, Johnson JL. Osteomyelitis in diabetic foot ulcers. Prompt diagnosis can avert amputation. Postgrad Med 2005;118:11–5.

[7] Williams DT, Hilton JR, Harding KG. Diagnosing foot infection in diabetes. Clin Infect Dis 2004; 39(Suppl 2):S83–6.

[8] Armstrong DG, Lavery LA, Sariaya M, et al. Leukocytosis is a poor indicator of acute osteomyelitis of the foot in diabetes mellitus. J Foot Ankle Surg 1996;35:280–3.

[9] Eneroth M, Apelqvist J, Stenstrom A. Clinical characteristics and outcome in 223 diabetic patients with deep foot infections. Foot Ankle Int 1997;18:716–22.

[10] Berendt AR, Lipsky B. Is this bone infected or not? Differentiating neuro-osteoarthropathy from osteomyelitis in the diabetic foot. Curr Diab Rep 2004;4:424–9.

[11] Newman LG, Waller J, Palestro CJ, et al. Leukocyte scanning with 111In is superior to magnetic resonance imaging in diagnosis of clinically unsuspected osteomyelitis in diabetic foot ulcers. Diabetes Care 1992;15:1527–30.

[12] Nardone DA. Probing to bone in infected pedal ulcers. JAMA 1995;274:869–70.

[13] Sommer TC, Lee TH. Charcot foot: the diagnostic dilemma. Am Fam Physician 2001;64:1591–8.

[14] Bonakdar-pour A, Gaines VD. The radiology of osteomyelitis. Orthop Clin North Am 1983;14: 21–37.

[15] Schweitzer ME, Morrison WB. MR imaging of the diabetic foot. Radiol Clin North Am 2004;42: 61–71.

[16] Sella EJ, Grosser DM. Imaging modalities of the diabetic foot. Clin Podiatr Med Surg 2003;20: 729–40.

[17] Zhuang H, Sam JW, Chacko TK, et al. Rapid normalization of osseous FDG uptake following traumatic or surgical fractures. Eur J Nucl Med Mol Imaging 2003;30:1096–103.

[18] Johnson JE, Kennedy EJ, Shereff MJ, et al. Prospective study of bone, indium-111-labeled white blood cell, and gallium-67 scanning for the evaluation of osteomyelitis in the diabetic foot. Foot Ankle Int 1996;17:10–6.

[19] Yuh WT, Corson JD, Baraniewski HM, et al. Osteomyelitis of the foot in diabetic patients: evaluation with plain film, 99mTc-MDP bone scintigraphy, and MR imaging. AJR Am J Roentgenol 1989;152:795–800.

[20] Keenan AM, Tindel NL, Alavi A. Diagnosis of pedal osteomyelitis in diabetic patients using current scintigraphic techniques. Arch Intern Med 1989;149:2262–6.

[21] Nelson HT, Taylor A. Bone scanning in the diagnosis of acute osteomyelitis. Eur J Nucl Med 1980;5:267–9.

[22] Larcos G, Brown ML, Sutton RT. Diagnosis of osteomyelitis of the foot in diabetic patients: value of 111In-leukocyte scintigraphy. AJR Am J Roentgenol 1991;157:527–31.

[23] Seabold JE, Flickinger FW, Kao SC, et al. Indium-

111-leukocyte/technetium-99m-MDP bone and magnetic resonance imaging: difficulty of diagnosing osteomyelitis in patients with neuropathic osteoarthropathy. J Nucl Med 1990;31:549–56.

[24] Alazraki N, Dries D, Datz F, et al. Value of a 24-hour image (four-phase bone scan) in assessing osteomyelitis in patients with peripheral vascular disease. J Nucl Med 1985;26:711–7.

[25] Israel O, Gips S, Jerushalmi J, et al. Osteomyelitis and soft-tissue infection: differential diagnosis with 24 hour/4 hour ratio of Tc-99m MDP uptake. Radiology 1987;163:725–6.

[26] Rosenthall L. Radionuclide investigation of osteomyelitis. Curr Opin Radiol 1992;4:62–9.

[27] Blume PA, Dey HM, Daley LJ, et al. Diagnosis of pedal osteomyelitis with Tc-99m HMPAO labeled leukocytes. J Foot Ankle Surg 1997;36:120–6 [discussion: 160].

[28] Palestro CJ, Mehta HH, Patel M, et al. Marrow versus infection in the Charcot joint: indium-111 leukocyte and technetium-99m sulfur colloid scintigraphy. J Nucl Med 1998;39:346–50.

[29] King AD, Peters AM, Stuttle AW, et al. Imaging of bone infection with labelled white blood cells: role of contemporaneous bone marrow imaging. Eur J Nucl Med 1990;17:148–51.

[30] Craig JG, Amin MB, Wu K, et al. Osteomyelitis of the diabetic foot: MR imaging-pathologic correlation. Radiology 1997;203:849–55.

[31] Erdman WA, Tamburro F, Jayson HT, et al. Osteomyelitis: characteristics and pitfalls of diagnosis with MR imaging. Radiology 1991;180:533–9.

[32] Lipman BT, Collier BD, Carrera GF, et al. Detection of osteomyelitis in the neuropathic foot: nuclear medicine, MRI and conventional radiography. Clin Nucl Med 1998;23:77–82.

[33] Morrison WB, Schweitzer ME, Wapner KL, et al. Osteomyelitis in feet of diabetics: clinical accuracy, surgical utility, and cost-effectiveness of MR imaging. Radiology 1995;196:557–64.

[34] Marcus CD, Ladam-Marcus VJ, Leone J, et al. MR imaging of osteomyelitis and neuropathic osteoarthropathy in the feet of diabetics. Radiographics 1996;16:1337–48.

[35] Morrison WB, Ledermann HP. Work-up of the diabetic foot. Radiol Clin North Am 2002;40:1171–92.

[36] Vesco L, Boulahdour H, Hamissa S, et al. The value of combined radionuclide and magnetic resonance imaging in the diagnosis and conservative management of minimal or localized osteomyelitis of the foot in diabetic patients. Metabolism 1999;48:922–7.

[37] Morrison WB, Schweitzer ME, Batte WG, et al. Osteomyelitis of the foot: relative importance of primary and secondary MR imaging signs. Radiology 1998;207:625–32.

[38] Chacko TK, Zhuang H, Nakhoda KZ, et al. Applications of fluorodeoxyglucose positron emission tomography in the diagnosis of infection. Nucl Med Commun 2003;24:615–24.

[39] Ledermann HP, Morrison WB, Schweitzer ME. MR image analysis of pedal osteomyelitis: distribution, patterns of spread, and frequency of associated ulceration and septic arthritis. Radiology 2002;223:747–55.

[40] Zhuang H, Yu JQ, Alavi A. Applications of fluorodeoxyglucose-PET imaging in the detection of infection and inflammation and other benign disorders. Radiol Clin North Am 2005;43:121–34.

[41] Stumpe KD, Zanetti M, Weishaupt D, et al. FDG positron emission tomography for differentiation of degenerative and infectious endplate abnormalities in the lumbar spine detected on MR imaging. AJR Am J Roentgenol 2002;179:1151–7.

[42] Temmerman OP, Heyligers IC, Hoekstra OS, et al. Detection of osteomyelitis using FDG and positron emission tomography. J Arthroplasty 2001;16:243–6.

[43] Zhuang H, Duarte PS, Pourdehnad M, et al. The promising role of 18F-FDG PET in detecting infected lower limb prosthesis implants. J Nucl Med 2001;42:44–8.

[44] Stumpe KD, Dazzi H, Schaffner A, et al. Infection imaging using whole-body FDG-PET. Eur J Nucl Med 2000;27:822–32.

[45] Ichiya Y, Kuwabara Y, Sasaki M, et al. A clinical evaluation of FDG-PET to assess the response in radiation therapy for bronchogenic carcinoma. Ann Nucl Med 1996;10:193–200.

[46] Stumpe KD, Notzli HP, Zanetti M, et al. FDG PET for differentiation of infection and aseptic loosening in total hip replacements: comparison with conventional radiography and three-phase bone scintigraphy. Radiology 2004;231:333–41.

[47] Ichiya Y, Kuwabara Y, Sasaki M, et al. FDG-PET in infectious lesions: the detection and assessment of lesion activity. Ann Nucl Med 1996;10:185–91.

[48] Kalicke T, Schmitz A, Risse JH, et al. Fluorine-18 fluorodeoxyglucose PET in infectious bone diseases: results of histologically confirmed cases. Eur J Nucl Med 2000;27:524–8.

[49] Zhuang H, Duarte PS, Pourdehand M, et al. Exclusion of chronic osteomyelitis with F-18 fluorodeoxyglucose positron emission tomographic imaging. Clin Nucl Med 2000;25:281–4.

[50] Zhuang H, Alavi A. 18-Fluorodeoxyglucose positron emission tomographic imaging in the detection and monitoring of infection and inflammation. Semin Nucl Med 2002;32:47–59.

[51] Sahlmann CO, Siefker U, Lehmann K, et al. Dual time point 2-[18F]fluoro-2'-deoxyglucose positron emission tomography in chronic bacterial osteomyelitis. Nucl Med Commun 2004;25:819–23.

[52] Keidar Z, Militianu D, Melamed E, et al. The diabetic foot: initial experience with 18F-FDG PET/CT. J Nucl Med 2005;46:444–9.

[53] Hopfner S, Krolak C, Kessler S, et al. Preoperative imaging of Charcot neuroarthropathy in diabetic patients: comparison of ring PET, hybrid PET,

and magnetic resonance imaging. Foot Ankle Int 2004;25:890–5.

[54] Cheung MHJ, Reddy S, Newberg A, et al. Diagnostic accuracy of FDG-PET imaging in detecting osteomyelitis of the diabetic foot. J Nucl Med 2005;46:134–5.

[55] Zhuang HM, Cortes-Blanco A, Pourdehnad M, et al. Do high glucose levels have differential effect on FDG uptake in inflammatory and malignant disorders? Nucl Med Commun 2001;22: 1123–8.

[56] Koort JK, Makinen TJ, Knuuti J, et al. Comparative 18F-FDG PET of experimental Staphylococcus aureus osteomyelitis and normal bone healing. J Nucl Med 2004;45:1406–11.

[57] Alnafisi N, Yun M, Alavi A. F-18 FDG positron emission tomography to differentiate diabetic osteoarthropathy from septic arthritis. Clin Nucl Med 2001;26:638–9.

[58] Makinen TJ, Lankinen P, Poyhonen T, et al. Comparison of (18)F-FDG and (68)Ga PET imaging in the assessment of experimental osteomyelitis due to Staphylococcus aureus. Eur J Nucl Med Mol Imaging 2005;32:1259–68.

[59] Brunner M, Langer O, Dobrozemsky G, et al. [18F]Ciprofloxacin, a new positron emission tomography tracer for noninvasive assessment of the tissue distribution and pharmacokinetics of ciprofloxacin in humans. Antimicrob Agents Chemother 2004;48:3850–7.

[60] Langer O, Brunner M, Zeitlinger M, et al. In vitro and in vivo evaluation of [18F]ciprofloxacin for the imaging of bacterial infections with PET. Eur J Nucl Med Mol Imaging 2005;32:143–50.

[61] Pellegrino D, Bonab AA, Dragotakes SC, et al. Inflammation and infection: imaging properties of 18F-FDG-labeled white blood cells versus 18F-FDG. J Nucl Med 2005;46:1522–30.

[62] Makinen TJ, Veiranto M, Knuuti J, et al. Efficacy of bioabsorbable antibiotic containing bone screw in the prevention of biomaterial-related infection due to Staphylococcus aureus. Bone 2005;36:292–9.

[63] Koch CJ, Hahn SM, Rockwell Jr K, et al. Pharmacokinetics of EF5 [2-(2-nitro-1-H-imidazol-1-yl)-N-(2,2,3,3,3-pentafluoropropyl) acetamide] in human patients: implications for hypoxia measurements in vivo by 2-nitroimidazoles. Cancer Chemother Pharmacol 2001;48:177–87.

[64] Gronroos T, Eskola O, Lehtio K, et al. Pharmacokinetics of [18F]FETNIM: a potential marker for PET. J Nucl Med 2001;42:1397–404.

[65] Evans SM, Kachur AV, Shiue CY, et al. Noninvasive detection of tumor hypoxia using the 2-nitroimidazole [18F]EF1. J Nucl Med 2000;41: 327–36.

[66] Evans SM, Hahn SM, Magarelli DP, et al. Hypoxia in human intraperitoneal and extremity sarcomas. Int J Radiat Oncol Biol Phys 2001;49: 587–96.

[67] Evans SM, Hahn S, Pook DR, et al. Detection of hypoxia in human squamous cell carcinoma by EF5 binding. Cancer Res 2000;60:2018–24.

[68] Dolbier Jr WR, Li AR, Koch CJ, et al. [18F]-EF5, a marker for PET detection of hypoxia: synthesis of precursor and a new fluorination procedure. Appl Radiat Isot 2001;54:73–80.

[69] Barthel H, Wilson H, Collingridge DR, et al. In vivo evaluation of [18F]fluoroetanidazole as a new marker for imaging tumour hypoxia with positron emission tomography. Br J Cancer 2004;90:2232–42.

[70] Ziemer LS, Evans SM, Kachur AV, et al. Noninvasive imaging of tumor hypoxia in rats using the 2-nitroimidazole 18F-EF5. Eur J Nucl Med Mol Imaging 2003;30:259–66.

ELSEVIER
SAUNDERS

POSITRON
EMISSION
TOMOGRAPHY

PET Clin 1 (2006) 131–139

PET Imaging of Arthritis

Roland Hustinx, MD, PhD[a],*, Michel G. Malaise, MD, PhD[b]

- Isotopic imaging of arthritis
- Clinical studies with fluorodeoxyglucose PET
- Methodologic considerations
- Imaging arthritis in the clinical setting
- Osteoarthritis
- Summary
- References

Inflammatory joint diseases include a wide variety of ailments, most of which are associated with an imbalance of the immune system. In this review, we focus on rheumatoid arthritis (RA), which is by far the most frequent, because it affects close to 1% of the population [1]. It is an autoimmune disease characterized by chronic inflammation of the synovium. Rheumatoid synovitis shows heavy leukocyte infiltrate, with neovascularization and proliferation of the synovial membrane. The inflamed and hypertrophic synovium is called the pannus, and it is directly responsible for the end result of the disease in the joints (cartilage and bone destruction). RA is a systemic disease, and it may affect many other organs. Without appropriate treatment, the disability may be high and mortality is significant. Major progress has been made in the understanding of and therapeutic approach to RA over the past 10 years. Potential treatments include anti-inflammatory drugs, nonsteroidal or steroidal, and disease-modifying antirheumatic drugs (DMARDs), with the latter being able to retard or stop the progression of the disease. These DMARDs are further classified into synthetic DMARDs, such as methotrexate, and biologic DMARDs, which were more recently developed, as well as target cytokines, such as tumor necrosis factor-α (TNFα) or interleukin-1

[2]. The advent of these biologic DMARDs has deeply modified the management and outcome of RA.

Left unchecked, the pannus is responsible for irreversible changes in the joints, which are visible on planar radiographs as joint space narrowing and marginal erosions. It is well recognized that an early diagnosis of the disease is of primary importance. Indeed, bone erosions occur early in the course of the disease, because radiographs show such modifications in 30% of the patients at the time of diagnosis and in 60% 2 years later [3]. Conversely, combinations of DMARDs are effective for preventing a long-term negative outcome [2]. This goal may only be achieved when treatment is initiated early after the onset of the disease. Obtaining such an early diagnosis is not an easy task, however, because many other diseases may mimic RA, at least at some stage of their course. In addition, the diagnostic criteria that are currently favored by the American College of Rheumatology rely heavily on clinical signs and symptoms, although they also include biologic testing of C-reactive protein (CRP) and radiographic changes. This approach may significantly delay appropriate patient management, because the clinical signs must be present for 6 weeks before the

[a] Division of Nuclear Medicine, University Hospital of Liège, University of Liège, Center of Cell and Molecular Therapy, Campus du Sart Tilman B35, Liège 4000, Belgium
[b] Division of Rheumatology, University Hospital of Liège, University of Liège, Center of Cell and Molecular Therapy, Campus du Sart Tilman B35, Liège 4000, Belgium
* Corresponding author.
E-mail address: rhustinx@chu.ulg.ac.be (R. Hustinx).

1556-8598/06/$ – see front matter © 2006 Elsevier Inc. All rights reserved.
pet.theclinics.com

doi:10.1016/j.cpet.2006.02.003

diagnosis is accepted and radiograph changes are often mere witnesses of irreversible damage. Newer approaches are therefore being investigated, taking advantage of technical developments in the field of imaging, particularly ultrasonography (US) and MRI [4].

Once limited to large joints, US equipped with newer high-frequency transducers is now able to image changes occurring in the small joints of the hands and feet. Synovial thickness can be accurately measured, and it has been shown to reflect synovitis. Furthermore, Doppler US detects increased blood flow in diseased joints, and the signal is correlated with microvascular synovial density, at least in large joints. Extra-articular structures, such as tendons and ligaments, are also easily evaluated. In addition, US can visualize bone erosions, at least in small accessible joints, such as the interphalangeal or metatarsophalangeal joints. US does not penetrate bone, however, which renders many joints inaccessible to the US evaluation of cartilage and bone surface [4]. These structures are better assessed using MRI, which, in fact, can visualize all aspects of inflammatory changes in joints, including those affecting the synovial membrane, synovial fluid, cartilage, bone, tendons, and ligaments. Whereas US measures the synovial thickness, MRI measures the inflammatory load (ie, the volume of inflamed synovial membrane) based on the quantification of the increase in signal intensity after intravenous injection of gadolinium contrast agent. MRI is also more sensitive than radiographs for detecting bone erosions, and it can even detect bone marrow edema, which may be an early sign preceding actual bone erosion [4]. Despite a fast-growing amount of scientific data, these two techniques are still in their development phase. Each has its strengths and limitations, and there is clearly a place for alternative imaging methods, such as PET.

Isotopic imaging of arthritis

The role of nuclear medicine techniques in the management of patients with inflammatory arthritis has always been quite limited. Even though three-phase bone scanning may be used as a screening modality, especially in patients in need of whole-body evaluation [5], its usefulness does not extend much beyond the diagnosis [6]. Fluorodeoxyglucose (FDG) PET imaging has the opportunity to become a major player in this field. It presents several advantages over bone scintigraphy. FDG accumulates in activated leukocytes and proliferating fibroblasts, which are important constituents of the inflammatory pannus. As a result, PET is able to visualize the inflammatory process directly rather than the secondary changes that are detected

with bone scanning, such as hyperemia or increased bone remodeling. It should be noted, however, that the increased FDG uptake observed in inflammatory joints results from highly complex phenomena, in which neoangiogenesis, apoptosis, and hypoxia contribute to modulate the process. Nonetheless, the biologic target of FDG seems to be highly relevant when it comes to imaging inflammation. In addition, PET offers much better spatial resolution than planar scintigraphy and the capability of reproducibly quantifying the tracer uptake, and thus the pathologic process. The advent of PET-CT further enhances the performance of metabolic imaging because it allows for a precise location of the foci of increased activity. Indeed, in small joints, such as the interphalangeal joints or metacarpophalangeal joints (MCPs), it may be difficult to distinguish uptake related to muscle activity from true synovitis. CT scanning performed during the same procedure also provides its own array of diagnostic information, such as bone erosion.

Clinical studies with fluorodeoxyglucose PET

The use of FDG PET for imaging RA was first reported by Polisson and colleagues [7]. They demonstrated highly increased FDG uptake in inflammatory joints in 2 patients, paralleled by synovial volumes estimated with MRI. The metabolic and MRI abnormalities dramatically decreased when the studies were repeated after treatment with prednisone and methotrexate. The same group performed FDG-PET and gadolinium-enhanced MRI of the wrists in 12 patients with inflammatory arthritis, including 9 with RA and 3 with psoriasic arthritis [8]. All patients had active disease and were imaged with MRI at baseline, 2 weeks after treatment with a nonsteroidal anti-inflammatory drug (NSAID) or prednisone was initiated, and a third time after 12 to 14 weeks of treatment with low-dose methotrexate. PET was not performed in 1 patient, and the baseline PET study was not interpretable in another patient. Imaging studies involved the most active wrist only, and clinical assessment was performed at each time point. The analysis was based on the measurement of the volume of enhancing pannus (VEP) on MRI and the standardized uptake value (SUV) on the PET studies. The authors found strong correlations between the VEP and SUV among the various data sets (at baseline and on the second and third studies) as well as between the changes in the VEP and SUV over time (statistically significant between the first and third evaluations only). In addition, MRI and PET parameters were strongly associated with clinical measures like pain, tenderness, and swelling. There was no correlation between metabolic and MRI measurements and the treatment outcome according to the Paulus index, however, which combines six clinical parameters. These findings are important, because it is the first time that a strong relation was demonstrated between metabolic activity, detection of the pannus with MRI, and clinical parameters in patients with inflammatory joint diseases. The fact that the outcome was not related to the imaging findings may have several possible explanations. The series was limited and heterogeneous because it combined two different diseases in only 10 patients fully assessable by PET. Also, the methodology for assessing the outcome (ie, the Paulus index) has its own limitations. In a study primarily aimed at evaluating ^{11}C-choline PET findings, Roivainen and coworkers [9] found a similar relation between FDG-PET, which was also performed, MRI, and clinical findings in 10 patients with various inflammatory joint diseases.

In an attempt to evaluate the potential of FDG-PET imaging in RA further, our group conducted a series of clinical studies. We first studied 21 patients with active RA according to the criteria of the American College of Rheumatology [10]. All patients underwent comprehensive functional, clinical, and biologic evaluations, including the Health Assessment Questionnaire (HAQ), morning stiffness, the patient global assessment (PGA), the physician global assessment (PhyGA), the disease activity score (DAS$_{28}$), the simplified disease activity index (SDAI), and laboratory tests (eg, CRP, erythrocyte sedimentation rate [ESR], and IgM rheumatoid factor). In addition, US was performed to assess the synovial thickness. The knees were imaged in all patients; the wrists, MCPs, and proximal interphalangeal joints (PIPs) were measured in 13 patients; and the ankles and first metatarsophalangeal joints (MTP-1s) were measured in the 8 remaining patients. The choice of the hands or ankles and feet was based on the presence of clinical symptoms as reported by the patient. Overall, 360 joints were evaluated. PET images were first visually analyzed, with subsequent SUV measurements of all joints. Sixty-three percent of the joints were positive on PET, according to the visual analysis, which was lower than the number of clinically positive joints (75% were swollen and 79% were tender) but higher than the number of US-positive joints (56%). The SUV was significantly higher in diseased joints than in the normal ones. There were only 4 joints that were metabolically active but clinically and US-negative. Conversely, the proportion of PET-positive joints increased with the number of abnormal clinical and US parameters from 41% when only one parameter (swelling, tenderness, or increased synovial thickness on US) was present to 90% when all three parameters were present. A positive correlation was found between the synovial thickness and the SUV in all diseased joints, except the MTP-1. The best correlation was observed in the large joints (knees). Moreover, the number of positive joints according to the visual analysis and the cumulative SUV of all joints positive on PET were correlated with all the US, biologic, clinical, and functional parameters, except for the duration of morning stiffness and the HAQ results. These findings indicate that the metabolic activity of synovitis, as measured with PET, reflects the activity of the disease in RA patients.

Given the increasingly convincing data regarding MRI in RA, we wanted to compare PET and US with this technique in a single homogeneous cohort of patients. We therefore conducted a study in 16 patients with active RA, who were imaged before and 4 weeks after initiation of anti-TNFα treatment [11]. Only one joint per patient (one knee) could be evaluated, however, because dynamic MRI requires dedicated coils and the accessibility of the technique remains limited for that purpose. As expected, we found that PET positivity was strongly associated with positivity on MRI and US. Again, the SUVs were higher in PET-positive joints, as were the synovial thickness and the MRI parameters, such as the relative enhancement 30 seconds after gadolinium injection, the rate of early enhancement at 55 seconds, and the static enhancement 15 minutes after gadolinium injection. CRP and metalloprotease-3 (MMP-3) levels also tended to be higher in the PET-positive joints, although the difference was not statistically significant. These values were significantly correlated with the SUVs, however, as well as with the synovial thickness, but only the dynamic MRI parameters were correlated with MMP-3 levels and not with CRP. These findings are yet additional proof that PET measurement of FDG uptake in inflamed joints is directly related to physiopathologic phenomena, as evidenced by other validated techniques. Interestingly enough, changes in SUVs were the only parameter correlated with changes in CRP and MMP-3 levels after anti-TNFα treatment. This is encouraging in the perspective of using PET as a method for quantifying the response to treatment early on, and perhaps for predicting the outcome.

Methodologic considerations

Several issues require clarification before even considering the performance of large trials with PET in inflammatory joint diseases. The kinetics of FDG uptake are relatively well known in cancer. In most tumors, the uptake increases over time for several hours before eventually reaching a plateau [12–14]. In contrast, such a plateau is reached fairly early on after tracer injection in benign tumors [15]. Dual time-point imaging with delayed studies also indicates that the uptake in inflammatory lesions remains stable over time [16]. Conversely, animal experiments with a turpentine-induced inflammation model showed that the uptake increases over 60 minutes after injection and then gradually decreases over time [17]. Little is known regarding the early phase of FDG uptake in the inflamed synovium, however. An initial portion of the answer was provided in the study by Roivainen and coworkers [9]. As dynamic acquisitions were performed in 2 patients, data revealed that the uptake in the pannus is initially fast but that it reaches a plateau early on, approximately 10 minutes after injection, and remains stable for the ensuing 50 minutes. We performed dynamic FDG-PET acquisitions in 17 patients with active psoriatic arthritis [18]. The imaging sequence was as follows: 13 2-minute frames started 2 minutes after injection, 2 3-minute frames started 40 minutes after injection, and 1 3-minute frame started 75 minutes after injection. Thirteen knees in 9 patients displayed a typical visual pattern of synovitis and were used for the SUV analysis. In most knees, the uptake reached a plateau 16 minutes after injection, and in 4 knees, the peak activity was observed on the first frame 2 minutes after injection. It then slightly decreased until the 10th minute after injection. Delayed scans did not show any difference in uptake compared with the values obtained once the plateau is reached. These results suggest that the synovial uptake may show two distinct patterns during the initial phase after injection but that it remains stable for a prolonged period in all cases. Practically, this means that arthritis patients may be imaged earlier than cancer patients (ie, 30 minutes after injection), which may be an asset when throughput is an issue.

Because published clinical data are still limited, the optimal methodology for interpreting the studies is not fully defined. A typical pattern of synovitis is easily recognized on the PET images and may thus objectify joint inflammation and orientate the diagnosis toward RA. Quantitative measurements are desired to assess the activity of the disease, however, and its response to treatment. Therefore, each question that is still subject to debate in the field of oncologic PET imaging is also relevant for arthritis imaging. In particular, whether the SUV would be good enough a parameter is likely but not fully established. Furthermore, the question of which normalization (body weight, body surface area, or lean body mass) should be preferred for calculating the SUV has to be answered. There are indications that FDG uptake by inflammatory lesions is more influenced by blood glucose level than cancer cells [19]. In particular, glucose loading decreased the expression of the GLUT-1 transporters in noninfectious inflammatory lesions in a rat model [20]. It may therefore be critical to correct for blood glucose level, even though normalizing the SUV to a 100-mg/dL blood glucose level, as usually applied in oncology, seems to be far from satisfactory from a theoretic standpoint.

A potentially important limitation of PET is related to its limited spatial and anatomic resolutions. This is not really an issue regarding large joints, such as the knees, but it may be difficult to identify synovitis in small joints of the hands or feet. Indeed, these patients most often also have inflammation of the tendon sheaths, which may be mistaken for the pannus itself. The same problem may arise when high muscular uptake is observed. In spite of this, we and others have observed low intra- and extraobserver coefficients of variation. The visual identification of the synovitis pattern was obtained with κ-values of 0.90 and 0.82 (intraobserver and extraobserver variability, respectively) [10]. For measuring the SUVs, the intraobserver coefficient of variation was 3.9%. The extraobserver coefficient was slightly higher at 14.9% and was directly related to the type of joints. A perfect agreement was found in the knees, but the variability reached 23% in the MCPs. It is worth mentioning that these results were obtained with a now outdated PET device and without the help of the CT information. Palmer and colleagues [8] obtained similarly high interobserver agreement values. These data indicate that at least in the context of a prospective study, the inflamed synovium may be reproducibly quantified. Nonetheless, reading such studies is a tedious and time-consuming process, and it remains to be shown that such high reproducibility can be reached in the clinical setting. PET-CT should largely address this issue because it provides precise anatomic landmarks and greatly facilitates the interpretation of the images as well as the positioning of the regions of interest. Two examples are shown in **Figs. 1 and 2**. To contribute to the diagnostic information fully, the CT scan should be acquired with the appropriate parameters in terms of dose and collimation, possibly with intravenous contrast agents. Whether such a diagnostic CT scan is needed in addition to or in place of the low-dose CT scan is yet another open question. Because inflammatory joint diseases often strike young patients, dosimetry has to be taken into account. Using low-dose CT and injecting FDG at a dose of 222 to 370 MBq, we obtain good-quality images while keeping the equiva-

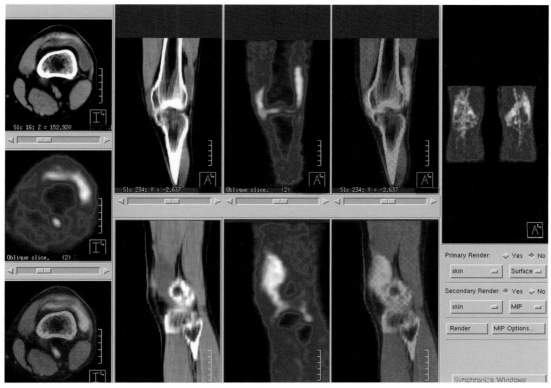

Fig. 1. Typical aspect of synovitis in both knees. The CT, PET, and fused images are shown in all three planes as well as the three-dimensional projection image of the PET study.

lent dose in the range of 8 to 12 mSv, which is acceptable [21].

Imaging arthritis in the clinical setting

The role of PET remains largely hypothetic at this stage, given the paucity of the available data. Nonetheless, there are several areas in which it may make a difference compared with other techniques. In the diagnosis of RA, PET would only be useful if it could detect inflammatory changes more reliably or earlier than other techniques. US and MRI are highly effective at detecting these changes; however, each has limitations. High-resolution contrast-enhanced MRI requires the appropriate coils and is limited to defined areas of the body. For instance, if one is to evaluate the knees and hands in one patient, the procedure would require four distinct acquisitions with two different coils. The acquisition and interpretation of MRI studies are time-consuming. Cost and availability are also issues, just as they are with PET. US, conversely, is widely available, relatively inexpensive, and, like MRI, has the advantage of not using ionizing radiation. As discussed previously, not all joints are accessible to

US, and, more importantly, it is highly operator dependent. It is unlikely that any of these limitations would prevent US and MRI from becoming useful clinical tools in the diagnosis and management of RA, however. PET may provide some answers to these shortcomings. It is quantitative and fairly reproducible, and it has the capability to image a large number of joints during a single session. With increased availability and improved throughput, overall cost is also decreasing. The major strength of PET stems from the fundaments of the signal being evaluated, that is, increased glucose metabolism in inflammatory tissues. Indeed, as pointed out by Brenner [22], increased synovial thickness and hypervascularization are morphology-based information. Only PET has the ability to provide molecular information regarding processes taking place at the cellular level.

Our understanding of the mechanism of FDG uptake in inflammatory lesions is growing, albeit it is still imperfect. Heelan and colleagues [23] studied two in vitro models of skin grafts. The FDG uptake was 1.5- to 2-fold higher in the allograft compared with the syngenic graft and was directly related to the extent of T-cell infiltrate. The type of cell taking up the tracer also varies

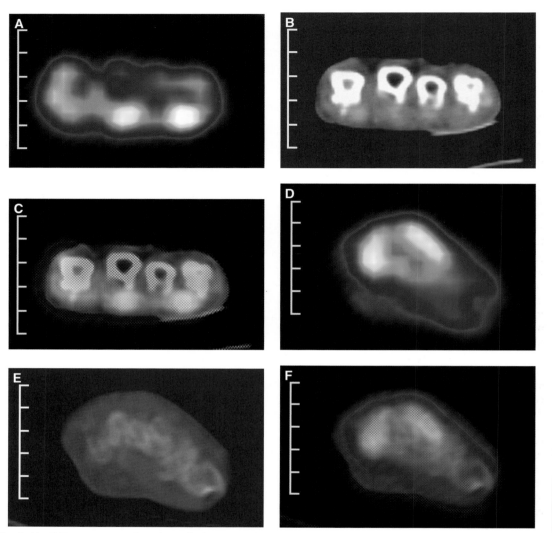

Fig. 2. (*A–C*) Transverse section through the MCPs shows tenosynovitis of the flexor muscles. (*D–F*) Transverse section through the wrist also shows synovitis of this joint.

depending on the inflammatory model: fibroblasts, endothelial cells, phagocytes, and, to a lesser extent, neutrophil polymorphonuclear and granulation tissues in turpentine-induced lesions [24]; T lymphocytes when selectively activated by concanavalin-A [25]; or B lymphocytes after viral infection in a monkey model [26]. More generally, the uptake is highest in activated inflammatory cells because of hyperexpression of glucose membrane transporters [27] and increased affinity of these transporters for glucose [28]. This phenomenon has not been described in tumor models. In neutrophils, the high increase in glucose metabolism precedes the respiratory burst and may be associated with the phenomenon of priming [29]. FDG-PET thus seems to be particularly well suited for studying the changes that occur in the inflamed joints. Pathologic examination of RA joints indeed reveals the accumulation of various cell lines in the synovial membrane: the synovial sublining layer contains macrophages, B and T lymphocytes, dendritic cells, and polymorphonuclear cells [30]. Macrophages and fibroblast-like synoviocytes are seen in the lining layer. The pannus-cartilage interface contains activated macrophages and synoviocytes. These cells secrete proteases, such as the matrix metalloproteases, which leads to cartilage loss and subsequent bone erosion. Other remarkable phenomena are the activation of osteoclasts and neoangiogenesis, which is essential for the proliferating pannus to invade the cartilage further. These cell populations and these pathologic phenomena are all associated with highly increased glucose metabolism. Moreover, the normal cartilage and the cartilage-bone interface do not show any significant FDG uptake under normal conditions, which is theoretically highly favorable to FDG-PET in terms of signal-to-noise ratio and, in all likelihood, specificity.

The potential role of PET as a diagnostic tool of early-stage RA remains to be evaluated. To date, it is not clear whether it presents any significant advantage over US and MRI, which are further advanced in their clinical validation process. PET is more likely to show an impact as a staging and treatment monitoring tool. Indeed, its whole-body capability should allow for an accurate determination of the number of inflamed joints, including the small ones. With PET-CT, tenosynovitis and bursitis can be identified. In addition to the extent of the disease, PET may quantify the intensity of uptake, which is directly related to the activity of the disease. The cumulative SUV or an index combining the cumulative SUV with the number of positive joints may well turn out to present unique prognostic value. In oncology, there are indications that high tumor SUVs are associated with poor prognosis [31–33]. The prognostic impact of the SUVs is still debated [34,35], however, and has yet to find a definite role in the treatment algorithms of cancer. In our series, we found a correlation between the SUVs and the presence of a Doppler signal, which is a sign of hypervascularization. Aggressive synovitis is known to present high levels of neovascularization. Because RA is a heterogenous disease, with many possible courses and outcomes that are unpredictable based on current diagnostic tests, it would be of tremendous value to identify early on the aggressive variants so as to tailor treatment on an individual basis [36]. In rheumatic diseases, as in oncology, only prospective longitudinal studies can answer this question. Nonetheless and regardless of any prognostic value, a baseline evaluation of disease activity is needed to assess the response to treatment early on. As mentioned previously, the trend is to treat aggressively with biologic DMARDs as soon as possible to limit the long-term negative effects of the disease [2]. These treatments are expensive and may result in serious side effects. In a limited series, we found that changes in SUVs measured as early as 4 weeks after administration of anti-TNFα were correlated with changes in MMP-3 levels [11]. Neither MRI nor US changes showed such a correlation. Because MMP-3 levels directly reflect the amount of inflamed synovium [37], this observation is a first important step toward using PET in the early assessment of therapeutic response. A reduction in synovial thickness at US is observed after successful treatment with anti-TNFα; however, this is seen only when US is performed later, after 6 to 18 weeks of treatment [38]. An example of the response to treatment is illustrated in Fig. 3.

Osteoarthritis

Osteoarthritis is a degenerative joint disorder, but it may present with highly active inflammatory phases. Wandler and coworkers [39] recently correlated PET findings in oncology patients with clinical syndromes of osteoarthritis. Fourteen of 21 patients with abnormal FDG uptake in the shoulder had a specific clinical diagnosis. In particular, 8 of 10 patients with diffuse uptake had osteoarthritis or bursitis. PET may also be of value to evaluate inflammation in osteoarthritis. The contribution of synovitis in this disease remains controversial. Investigators at the University of Pennsylvania observed increased FDG uptake in the synovium of 8 of 15 patients with proven degenerative disorders of the knees [40]. Further studies are needed of course, but the potential is there for PET, given the burden of osteoarthritis in health care.

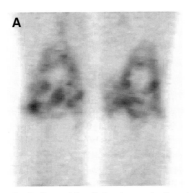 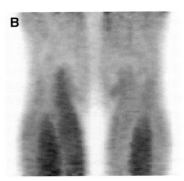

Fig. 3. Synovitis of the knees before (*A*) and 4 weeks after (*B*) treatment with infliximab.

Summary

FDG-PET imaging of arthritis is still in its infancy. Neither the optimal methodology nor the real clinical value is known at this time. Nevertheless, initial results are highly encouraging. The feasibility of the technique is demonstrated. PET findings are correlated with results obtained with state-of-the-art MRI and US as well as with established clinical assessment of RA. There are indications that FDG-PET may provide unique information regarding the prognosis and early response to treatment. The mechanism of FDG uptake in the diseased joints has to be clarified further, but the available data indicate that it is well suited for imaging inflammatory joint disorders and, possibly, osteoarthritis. What lies ahead is the important work of clinical validation to verify the diagnostic and prognostic accuracy before envisioning a clinical role in routine practice.

References

[1] Scott DL, Symmons DP, Coulton BL, et al. Long-term outcome of treating rheumatoid arthritis: results after 20 years. Lancet 1987;1(8542): 1108–11.

[2] O'Dell JR. Therapeutic strategies for rheumatoid arthritis [see comment]. N Engl J Med 2004; 350(25):2591–602.

[3] van der Heijde DM. Joint erosions and patients with early rheumatoid arthritis. Br J Rheumatol 1995;34(Suppl 2):74–8.

[4] Ostergaard M, Ejbjerg B, Szkudlarek M. Imaging in early rheumatoid arthritis: roles of magnetic resonance imaging, ultrasonography, conventional radiography and computed tomography. Best Pract Res Clin Rheumatol 2005;19(1): 91–116.

[5] Backhaus M, Burmester GR, Sandrock D, et al. Prospective two year follow up study comparing novel and conventional imaging procedures in patients with arthritic finger joints. Ann Rheum Dis 2002;61(10):895–904.

[6] Fogelman I. Bone scanning. In: Maisey MN, Britton KE, Gilday DL, editors. Clinical nuclear medicine. London: Chapman and Hall Medical; 1991. p. 131–57.

[7] Polisson RP, Schoenberg OI, Fischman A, et al. Use of magnetic resonance imaging and positron emission tomography in the assessment of synovial volume and glucose metabolism in patients with rheumatoid arthritis. Arthritis Rheum 1995; 38(6):819–25.

[8] Palmer WE, Rosenthal DI, Schoenberg OI, et al. Quantification of inflammation in the wrist with gadolinium-enhanced MR imaging and PET with 2-[F-18]-fluoro-2-deoxy-D-glucose. Radiology 1995;196(3):647–55.

[9] Roivainen A, Parkkola R, Yli-Kerttula T, et al. Use of positron emission tomography with methyl-11C-choline and 2-18F-fluoro-2-deoxy-D-glucose in comparison with magnetic resonance imaging for the assessment of inflammatory proliferation of synovium. Arthritis Rheum 2003;48(11): 3077–84.

[10] Beckers C, Ribbens C, Andre B, et al. Assessment of disease activity in rheumatoid arthritis with (18)F-FDG PET. J Nucl Med 2004;45(6):956–64.

[11] Beckers C, Jeukens X, Ribbens C, et al. (18)F-FDG PET imaging of rheumatoid knee synovitis correlates with dynamic magnetic resonance and sonographic assessments as well as with the serum level of metalloproteinase-3. Eur J Nucl Med Mol Imaging 2006;33:245–80.

[12] Fischman AJ, Alpert NM. FDG-PET in oncology: there's more to it than looking at pictures. J Nucl Med 1993;34(1):6–11.

[13] Hamberg LM, Hunter GJ, Alpert NM, et al. The dose uptake ratio as an index of glucose metabolism: useful parameter or oversimplification? J Nucl Med 1994;35(8):1308–12.

[14] Boerner AR, Weckesser M, Herzog H, et al. Optimal scan time for fluorine-18 fluorodeoxyglucose positron emission tomography in breast cancer. Eur J Nucl Med 1999;26(3):226–30.

[15] Lodge MA, Lucas JD, Marsden PK, et al. PET study of 18FDG uptake in soft tissue masses. Eur J Nucl Med 1999;26(1):22–30.

[16] Hustinx R, Smith RJ, Benard F, et al. Dual time point fluorine-18 fluorodeoxyglucose positron emission tomography: a potential method to differentiate malignancy from inflammation and normal tissue in the head and neck. Eur J Nucl Med 1999;26(10):1345–8.

[17] Yamada S, Kubota K, Kubota R, et al. High accumulation of fluorine-18-fluorodeoxyglucose in turpentine-induced inflammatory tissue. J Nucl Med 1995;36(7):1301–6.

[18] Beckers C, Bernard C, Kaiser MJ, et al. Time-course study of FDG uptake in psoriasic synovitis. J Nucl Med 2005;46(Suppl 2):183P.

[19] Zhao S, Kuge Y, Tsukamoto E, et al. Effects of insulin and glucose loading on FDG uptake in experimental malignant tumours and inflammatory lesions. Eur J Nucl Med 2001;28(6):730–5.

[20] Zhao S, Kuge Y, Tsukamoto E, et al. Fluorodeoxyglucose uptake and glucose transporter expression in experimental inflammatory lesions and malignant tumours: effects of insulin and glucose loading. Nucl Med Commun 2002;23(6): 545–50.

[21] Brix G, Lechel U, Glatting G, et al. Radiation exposure of patients undergoing whole-body dual-modality 18F-FDG PET/CT examinations. J Nucl Med 2005;46(4):608–13.

[22] Brenner W. 18F-FDG PET in rheumatoid arthritis: there still is a long way to go [comment]. J Nucl Med 2004;45(6):927–9.

[23] Heelan BT, Osman S, Blyth A, et al. Use of 2-[18F]fluoro-2-deoxyglucose as a potential agent

in the prediction of graft rejection by positron emission tomography. Transplantation 1998;66(8):1101–3.

[24] Yamada S, Kubota K, Kubota R, et al. High accumulation of fluorine-18-fluorodeoxyglucose in turpentine-induced inflammatory tissue. J Nucl Med 1995;36(7):1301–6.

[25] Ishimori T, Saga T, Mamede M, et al. Increased (18)F-FDG uptake in a model of inflammation: concanavalin A-mediated lymphocyte activation. J Nucl Med 2002;43(5):658–63.

[26] Scharko AM, Perlman SB, Hinds PW, et al. Whole body positron emission tomography imaging of simian immunodeficiency virus-infected rhesus macaques. Proc Natl Acad Sci USA 1996;93(13): 6425–30.

[27] Gamelli RL, Liu H, He LK, et al. Augmentations of glucose uptake and glucose transporter-1 in macrophages following thermal injury and sepsis in mice. J Leukoc Biol 1996;59(5):639–47.

[28] Ahmed N, Kansara M, Berridge MV. Acute regulation of glucose transport in a monocyte-macrophage cell line: Glut-3 affinity for glucose is enhanced during the respiratory burst. Biochem J 1997;327(Pt 2):369–75.

[29] Jones HA, Cadwallader KA, White JF, et al. Dissociation between respiratory burst activity and deoxyglucose uptake in human neutrophil granulocytes: implications for interpretation of (18)F-FDG PET images. J Nucl Med 2002;43(5): 652–7.

[30] Paleolog EM. Angiogenesis in rheumatoid arthritis. Arthritis Res 2002;4(Suppl 3):S81–90.

[31] Sasaki R, Komaki R, Macapinlac H, et al. [18F] fluorodeoxyglucose uptake by positron emission tomography predicts outcome of non-small-cell lung cancer. J Clin Oncol 2005;23(6):1136–43.

[32] Borst GR, Belderbos JS, Boellaard R, et al. Standardised FDG uptake: a prognostic factor for inoperable non-small cell lung cancer. Eur J Cancer 2005;41(11):1533–41.

[33] Downey RJ, Akhurst T, Gonen M, et al. Preoperative F-18 fluorodeoxyglucose-positron emission tomography maximal standardized uptake value predicts survival after lung cancer resection. J Clin Oncol 2004;22(16):3255–60.

[34] Atkins CD. Overestimation of the prognostic significance of SUV measurement by positron emission tomography for non-small-cell lung cancer. J Clin Oncol 2005;23(27):6799–800.

[35] van Westreenen HL, Plukker JT, Cobben DC, et al. Prognostic value of the standardized uptake value in esophageal cancer. AJR Am J Roentgenol 2005;185(2):436–40.

[36] Landewe RB, van der Heijde DM. Early rheumatoid arthritis: toward tailor-made therapy. Curr Rheumatol Rep 2003;5(4):287–93.

[37] Ribbens C, Martin y Porras M, Franchimont N, et al. Increased matrix metalloproteinase-3 serum levels in rheumatic diseases: relationship with synovitis and steroid treatment. Ann Rheum Dis 2002;61(2):161–6.

[38] Taylor PC, Steuer A, Gruber J, et al. Comparison of ultrasonographic assessment of synovitis and joint vascularity with radiographic evaluation in a randomized, placebo-controlled study of infliximab therapy in early rheumatoid arthritis. Arthritis Rheum 2004;50(4):1107–16.

[39] Wandler E, Kramer EL, Sherman O, et al. Diffuse FDG shoulder uptake on PET is associated with clinical findings of osteoarthritis. AJR Am J Roentgenol 2005;185(3):797–803.

[40] El-Haddad G, Wolf M, Hochhold J, et al. The potential role of FDG-PET in the management of patients with osteoarthritic knees. J Nucl Med 2005;42(Suppl 2):182P.

ELSEVIER
SAUNDERS

POSITRON
EMISSION
TOMOGRAPHY

PET Clin 1 (2006) 141–152

Evaluating the Role of Fluorodeoxyglucose PET Imaging in the Management of Patients with Sarcoidosis

Jian Q. Yu, MD[a],*, Hongming Zhuang, MD, PhD[b], Ayse Mavi, MD[c], Abass Alavi, MD[c]

- ■ Conventional diagnostic imaging studies
  - Chest radiograph
  - CT scan
  - MRI
  - Conventional nuclear medicine methods
- ■ Role of PET for assessing sarcoidosis

- Pulmonary sarcoidosis
- Cardiac sarcoidosis
- Neurosarcoidosis
- Other organs
- ■ Summary
- ■ References

Sarcoidosis is a disorder of unknown etiology that affects individuals in different geographic locations and is characterized by the presence of multisystem noncaseating granulomas. It was first described by a dermatologist, Jonathan Hutchinson, in 1877, who reported his findings in a 50-year-old man who had large purple skin plaques on his hands and feet and in a 64-year-old woman with large purple patches on her face and arms [1]. Since this initial description, histopathologic characteristics of this disorder have been clearly defined and are the basis for making the diagnosis. This disease affects young adults more often than older subjects and generally presents with pulmonary manifestations; however, other organs and/or sys-

tems, including the skin, eyes, muscles, heart, and brain, can be affected initially or at later stages of the disease.

The exact prevalence of sarcoidosis is unknown. The incidence is different in various geographic locations around the world and in the United States, and it is more commonly noted in African-American populations than in the other ethnic groups [2]. It has been estimated that the lifetime risk of sarcoidosis in blacks in the United States is 2.4% compared with a lifetime risk of 0.85% in whites [3].

The exact cause and pathogenesis of sarcoidosis are not clear at the present time. The current and widely held hypotheses are that sarcoidosis has

[a] Department of Diagnostic Imaging, Fox Chase Cancer Center, 333 Cottman Avenue, Philadelphia, PA 19111, USA
[b] Division of Nuclear Medicine, Department of Radiology, The Children's Hospital of Philadelphia, 34th Street and Civic Center Boulevard, Philadelphia, PA 19104, USA
[c] Division of Nuclear Medicine, Department of Radiology, Hospital of the University of Pennsylvania, 110 Donner Building, 3400 Spruce Street, Philadelphia, PA 19104, USA
* Corresponding author.
E-mail address: michael.yu@fccc.edu (J.Q. Yu).

doi:10.1016/j.cpet.2006.01.002

pet.theclinics.com

multiple causes, which can explain the different patterns and manifestations of illness [4]. Assessment of disease activity by conventional imaging methods is difficult and unreliable; however, accurate determination of disease activity is essential for timely administration of corticosteroids to control the disease. The natural course of the disease in individual patients is quite variable. Sarcoidosis is self-limited in many patients; yet, a mortality rate of approximately 5% is associated with this disorder. For this review, we focus on the role of imaging modalities for the initial and follow-up assessment of sarcoidosis. Accurate assessment of the disease activity is of great clinical importance in the timely management of these patients.

Conventional diagnostic imaging studies

More than 90% of patients with sarcoidosis are detected by the abnormalities noted on conventional chest radiographs or CT scans of the thorax. Bilateral hilar adenopathy is the "classic" chest radiographic finding, but it is not specific for sarcoidosis. Parenchymal infiltrates seen in a segment of the population may be interstitial, alveolar, or both. Infrequently (<5% of patients), pleural involvement can result in lymphocytic exudative effusion, chylothorax, hemothorax, or pneumothorax.

Chest radiograph

The classification of pulmonary involvement in sarcoidosis is based on the radiographic stage of the disease:

Stage I: bilateral hilar adenopathy only. Fifty percent of affected patients exhibit bilateral hilar adenopathy as the first expression of sarcoidosis.
Stage II: bilateral hilar adenopathy and interstitial infiltrates (the latter occurs more often in the upper than in the lower lung zones). These findings are present at the initial diagnosis in 25% of the patients.
Stage III: interstitial disease with shrinking hilar nodes. Interstitial opacities are commonly present at this stage and are predominantly distributed in the upper lung zones.
Stage IV: advanced fibrosis of the lungs bilaterally

Additional pulmonary findings that can occur in patients with sarcoidosis include the following:

- Nodular opacities
- Endobronchial involvement in 40% of stage I patients and 70% of stage II and III patients
- Significant stenosis of the airways; this abnormality is uncommon and can cause significant morbidity when it is severe.

- Submucosal noncaseating epithelioid granulomas of the lower and upper airways, including the larynx, pharynx, and sinuses

Although the chest radiograph provides a useful anatomic guide for assessing lung involvement, it cannot determine disease activity and functional consequences of the inflammatory process in the affected sites. In general, chest radiographic findings are noted relatively late in the course of the disease, and monitoring the response to treatment is quite limited using this imaging technique.

CT scan

Tomographic images demonstrate a variety of abnormalities; overall, they are more accurate and sensitive than chest radiographs in assessing the presence and extent of the disease. The CT findings can be summarized as follows:

- Hilar and mediastinal lymphadenopathy
- Beaded or irregular thickening of the bronchovascular bundles
- Nodules along bronchi, vessels, and subpleural regions
- Bronchial wall thickening
- Ground-glass opacification
- Parenchymal masses or consolidation
- Parenchymal bands
- Cysts
- Traction bronchiectasis
- Fibrosis with distortion of the lung architecture

High-resolution CT (HRCT) scanning reveals the predominance of these changes in the middle to upper zones. It can also detect parenchymal abnormalities that are not seen on plain chest radiographs.

The HRCT findings correlate well with the histologic abnormalities. Ground-glass opacities, for example, are associated with sarcoid granulomas rather than with alveolitis. This finding has raised the question as to whether alveolitis is a prominent feature of sarcoidosis. Alveolitis is rarely identified in patients with clinically significant disease. A CT scan is useful for detecting recurrence, but the sensitivity of the technique is suboptimal for detecting early disease.

MRI

MRI is useful for suspected neurosarcoidosis, but its role in assessing pulmonary sarcoidosis is limited. MRI is also of value in detecting solid organ involvement by sarcoidosis.

Conventional nuclear medicine methods

Gallium-67 (Ga-67) scanning is one of the early studies used for the diagnosis and management of sarcoidosis [5]. This radiotracer localizes at the inflammatory sites in the lung but not in the normal parenchyma [6–8]. Whole-body gallium scanning has been used as a sensitive but nonspecific indicator of disease activity in other organs. It is particularly useful for the diagnosis of the disease in patients with normal chest radiographs and/or otherwise atypical presentations. Patterns of symmetrically increased uptake in the mediastinal and hilar nodes (λ) and in the lacrimal, parotid, and salivary glands (panda sign) are considered pathognomonic for sarcoidosis [Fig. 1]. Gallium scanning may guide the clinician to the appropriate biopsy sites and may help to determine whether radiologic densities represent reversible inflammation or fibrosis. Gallium uptake is affected by systemic administration of corticosteroids; thus, a negative scan in patients being treated with prednisone may be unreliable for detecting active disease. A negative study may indicate a favorable response to this drug, however.

It has been shown that there is a direct relation between a visual index of Ga-67 uptake in the lung and the number of inflammatory cells (particularly macrophages) recovered by bronchoalveolar lavage in patients with sarcoidosis (and idiopathic pulmonary fibrosis) [6–8]. Therefore, the degree of uptake of Ga-67 may be useful in determining the level of alveolar inflammation in these patients because the agent is primarily concentrated in the alveolar macrophages and, to a lesser degree, in the neutrophils. In addition, studies in normal subjects have demonstrated that a small but significant amount of Ga-67 in the alveolar macrophages obtained by bronchoalveolar lavage is detected despite negative pulmonary images [9,10].

Ga-67 lung scanning is not recommended for the routine evaluation of patients with suspected or known sarcoidosis. Ga-67 scanning has been accepted as a tool for monitoring the response to therapy for patients with positive baseline examinations [5]. A whole-body Ga-67 study is useful for detecting clinically silent sites for obtaining a tissue biopsy so as to secure a diagnosis [11]. In general, the study is difficult to interpret, the findings are nonspecific, and a negative scan does not exclude disease [12]. A Ga-67 scan can be used in clinical settings in which state-of-the-art imaging studies (eg, PET) are not available, however [11].

Thallium (Tl)-201 and technetium (Tc)-99m sestamibi imaging has been used to diagnose a cardiac sarcoid, differentiate it from coronary artery disease, and monitor the response to treatment. This is discussed in more detail elsewhere in the cardiac sarcoidosis section of this article.

In recent years, some newer radiotracers have been used for the diagnosis and assessment of patients with sarcoidosis [13,14]. In a prospective pilot study using Tc-99m–labeled depreotide in 22 patients with known sarcoidosis, it was shown that this agent binds to specific somatostatin receptors. Scans were positive in 18 patients (81%), and all 4 patients with negative scans had normal plain chest radiographs. In addition, the study demonstrated all sites of nonpulmonary lesions. The images correlated well with the disease stage as determined by chest radiographs and pulmonary func-

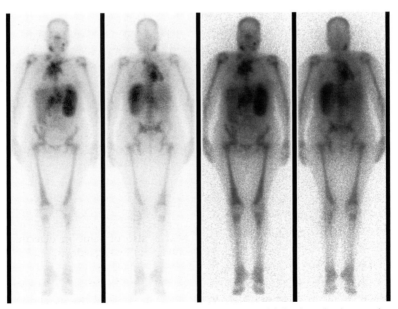

Fig. 1. Classic λ (lambda) in the chest attributable to mediastinal and hilar lymphadenopathy as shown in this planar Ga-67 whole-body scan. Note that the spleen is significantly enlarged and is affected by the disease.

tion tests; however, the role of this approach is unclear, and the compound is no longer available for clinical purposes in the United States.

In another study, results of Ga-67 scans and indium (In)-111–labeled pentetreotide scans were compared in patients with sarcoidosis. The latter tracer is a peptide that binds to the somatostatin receptors. The results showed the superiority of peptide imaging over Ga-67 scanning not only on a patient-by-patient basis (18 of 18 for peptide versus 16 of 18 for Ga-67) but on a lesion-by-lesion basis (64 of 99 for Ga-67 versus 82 of 99 for peptide). This head-to-head comparison demonstrates that somatostatin receptor imaging may prove to be superior to Ga-67 scanning in the management of these patients.

Role of PET for assessing sarcoidosis

PET, along with 18F-fluorodeoxyglucose (FDG), has been widely used for examining patients with cancer as well as cardiac and neurologic disorders.

In recent years, the role of FDG-PET imaging in the evaluation of inflammatory and infectious processes has been widely explored [15–22]. As an inflammatory disorder, sarcoidosis is an appropriate candidate for this powerful technique.

Pulmonary sarcoidosis

The first report of FDG-PET imaging in sarcoidosis appeared in the literature in 1987 [23]. In the early 1990s, another report described two cases of sarcoidosis with positive FDG-PET findings, which were erroneously interpreted to represent lymphoma [24]. Two editorials in the same issue of the journal projected a role for this methodology for the management of patients with this disorder [25,26]. These articles indicated that PET may not be a major tool for the initial diagnosis of sarcoidosis but that it may play a role in the management of the patients with this disorder. Since then, several case reports have been published in the literature and describe patients who were discovered incidentally to have a sarcoid by FDG-PET

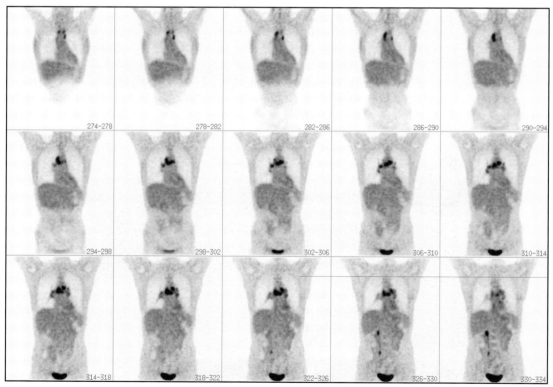

Fig. 2. This 43-year-old female patient with newly diagnosed invasive ductal right breast cancer underwent an FDG-PET examination for preoperative staging. The PET study revealed multiple foci of increased uptake in bilateral hilar, mediastinal, and paratracheal regions consistent with an FDG avid metabolically active process; the pattern of activity is not typical for breast cancer metastases and can be caused by conditions like lymphoma or sarcoidosis. Histopathologic examination of these lesions obtained from the mediastinoscopy demonstrated multiple fragments of lymph node with noncaseating granulomas and no malignant cells.

imaging [Fig. 2] [24,27,28]. In one case, recurrent sarcoidosis was discovered in the transplanted lungs [29]. Incidentally detected sarcoidosis has been interpreted as cancer in the setting of a work-up for a malignant disease [Figs. 3 and 4] [30,31].

Another case report revealed the superiority of FDG-PET over Ga-67 scanning for the diagnosis of this disease [32]. In this patient, the FDG-PET images showed extensive disease activity in the chest and brain, whereas the Ga-67 study was unremarkable. We examined 28 patients with 31 FDG-PET studies at various stages of the disease [15]. All patients had an established diagnosis or CT findings that were suggestive of sarcoidosis. The typical patterns on FDG-PET images were similar to those on the Ga-67 images and included bilateral hilar activity extending to the mediastinum and lung parenchyma. This was seen on 71% of the FDG-PET images in this series. The second observation demonstrated a significant discrepancy between PET and CT scans (6 of 31 [19%]); PET showed multiple foci of intense activity within and outside the chest, whereas CT showed only a solitary nod-ule. Activity in the spleen was seen commonly in this group of patients. Response to treatment was more clearly detected by PET than by CT. In 10% of this population, CT showed multiple small lesions in the lungs that were suggestive of metastases from an unknown primary tumor. FDG-PET showed a similar finding in the lungs and at no other site in the body. This discrepancy raised the possibility of an inflammatory process in the lungs, such as sarcoidosis, which was proven by further studies.

As noted previously and described in the literature [31–39], sarcoidosis can mimic malignant diseases, such as lymphomas and lung cancer. Dual-time or delayed imaging allows differentiating some benign lesions, such as inflammation, from malignant diseases [40–42]. There is no evidence that dual–time-point imaging might be useful in differentiating sarcoidosis from malignancy, however. In general, malignant lesions have more metabolic activity than benign disorders [39], but there is a considerable degree of overlap between the two [43]. As an inflammatory process, sarcoidosis is an exception to this

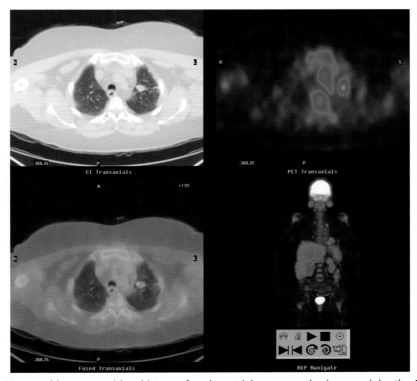

Fig. 3. In this 59-year-old woman with a history of endometrial cancer and a lung nodule, the PET-CT images demonstrated a nodule that seemed to be metabolically active with increased FDG uptake (*red in upper right image*). The upper left image is the corresponding CT image; the lower left image is the PET and CT fusion image, and the lower right image is the projection image of the body. These findings were reported to represent metastatic disease because of the patient's past history. The nodule was excised, and the pathologic examination revealed a granuloma.

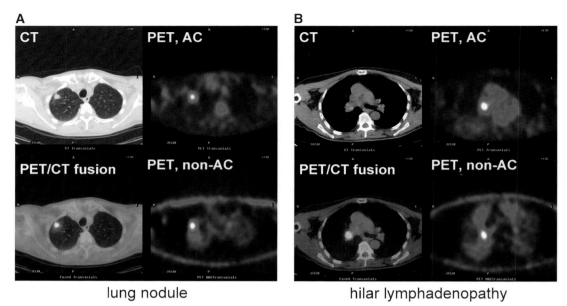

lung nodule   hilar lymphadenopathy

Fig. 4. This 70-year-old man has a spiculated right upper lung nodule and hilar lymphadenopathy. The PET-CT scan is positive for the nodule (A, CT in lung window) and lymph node (B, CT in mediastinal window), which is consistent with a metabolically active process (red/white color focus). A core biopsy was obtained and showed nonnecrotizing granulomas. AC, attenuation corrected.

observation and usually shows high metabolic activity at different stages of the disease [39,42,44].

Sarcoidosis can be diagnosed based on the typical and classic patterns of the uptake of FDG or other tracers [24,30]. Not infrequently, however, it can mimic malignant disorders; as such, it is a source of false-positive findings as noted in the published literature [28,42,45–55]. Some case reports describe positive findings after the induction of chemotherapy and radiation therapy [56,57]. Yao and colleagues [57] reported a patient who showed abnormal uptake in the neck and mediastinum after intensity-modulated radiation therapy (IMRT). The pretreatment PET scan was normal in the chest, and a biopsy showed granulomatous changes with necrosis.

Based on our own experience, FDG-PET scanning is quite valuable in evaluating pulmonary sarcoidosis as well as extrapulmonary involvement of the disease [Fig. 5] [16,32]. An FDG-PET scan is quite valuable in detecting unsuspected sites of involvement and leading to successful diagnosis and therapy. This technique is also of value in monitoring treatment response and in deciding whether to continue or switch to an alternate therapeutic regimen [Fig. 6].

Brudin and coworkers [33] have introduced a new concept for assessing regional pulmonary glucose metabolism (MRglu) as an index of the degree of inflammation and have related it to other tests, such as routine pulmonary function tests, chest ra-

diography, and serum angiotensin-converting enzyme (SACE) levels. MRglu was measured in a single midthoracic transaxial slice using PET in seven patients with histologically proven sarcoidosis before and after high-dose steroid therapy. The authors concluded that MRglu measured with FDG-PET may reflect "disease activity" in sarcoidosis in quantitative terms (per gram of lung tissue) and with respect to disease distribution. The utility of this approach should be verified and validated in a large population before adopting it on a routine basis.

Milman and colleagues [58] used FDG-PET to investigate temporal changes in disease activity in a patient with pulmonary sarcoidosis before and during therapy with inhaled corticosteroids, followed by systemic administration of this drug. FDG-PET was performed at baseline and then 10 and 14 months after treatment. Before the second PET scan, the patient was treated with an inhaled corticosteroid (beclomethasone), and before the third PET scan, the patient was treated with oral prednisolone. The first PET scan showed high FDG uptake in the hilar and mediastinal lymph nodes and in the pulmonary parenchyma and pleura. The second PET scan showed reduced uptake in the mediastinal lymph nodes, but there seemed to be no change in the lungs and the pleura. The third PET scan showed no evidence of active disease, however. They concluded that based on FDG-PET, inhaled cortico-

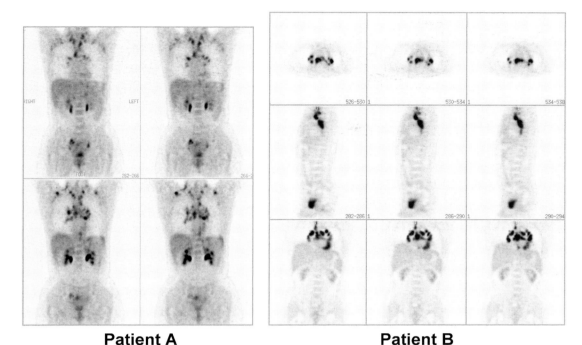

Patient A   **Patient B**

Fig. 5. Patient A: Coronal image set (two images in each row) on the left is the typical pattern of FDG uptake in a patient with sarcoidosis. Increased uptake is noted in the lymph nodes in the supraclavicular, mediastinal, and hilar regions bilaterally. Patient B: Image set on the right shows lymph nodes in the hilar and the mediastinal chain of another patient with sarcoidosis. These images are displayed in the transaxial (*top row*), sagittal (*middle row*), and coronal (*lower row*) views.

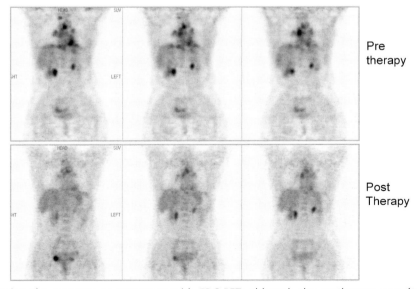

Fig. 6. Monitoring the response to treatment with FDG-PET; although the pretherapy scan (*top row*) show significant disease in the mediastinum, the posttherapy scan (*bottom row*) demonstrates marked improvement with significantly decreased metabolic activity at the sites of enlarged lymphadenopathy.

steroids had no recognizable influence on inflammatory disease activity. In contrast, treatment with oral prednisolone reduced disease activity, as demonstrated by PET. These data are concordant with clinical studies that show a marginal effect from inhaled corticosteroids and a marked response from the systemic administration of this drug. This study suggests that PET is a useful tool for testing the efficacy of various treatments and the optimal route of administering these drugs.

In addition to FDG, other PET tracers have been used to evaluate sarcoidosis and other granulomatous disease [59]. Halter and coworkers [60] studied the thymidine analogue 3-deoxy-3[(18)F]-fluorothymidine (FLT) and compared the results with those of FDG-PET scanning. FLT is a tracer that specifically targets the proliferative activity of malignant and noncancerous cells. This prospective study was performed during a preoperative workup, with subsequent pathologic correlations. The preliminary findings indicated that compared with FDG uptake, FLT uptake is specific for malignant lesions and reveals fewer false-positive findings in patients with sarcoidosis.

Yamada and colleagues [61] conducted a study in which carbon (C)-11–methionine (Met) was used to evaluate mediastinal and hilar lymph nodes in 31 patients with sarcoidosis. The study was designed to examine and define the role of FDG-PET and C-11–Met PET in the clinical assessment of pulmonary involvement with this disease. These scans were performed within a few days of each other. The differential uptake ratio of these tracers was calculated for the region of interest with the most intense activity. All patients had a minimum of 1 year of follow-up, which included a clinical reassessment. There were repeat studies for 7 patients in whom lymph nodes still remained visible on these imaging studies. These investigators also calculated the FDG/Met uptake ratios and divided patients into an FDG-dominant group (FDG/Met uptake ratio ≥ 2) and a Met-dominant group (FDG/Met uptake ratio < 2).

They noted that the rate of improvement assessed by clinical findings and chest radiographs correlated considerably better in the FDG-dominant group (78%) than in the Met-dominant group (33%). In the seven patients with repeated PET examinations, the FDG/Met uptake ratios were unchanged after 1 year. The authors concluded that the FDG/Met uptake ratio by PET studies may reflect the differential granulomatous state in this disorder.

Oriuchi and coworkers [62] compared the uptake of F-18-fluoro-methyl-tyrosine (FMT) and FDG in 10 patients with sarcoidosis and 10 patients with lung cancer so as to distinguish sarcoidosis from malignancy. Interestingly, they noted that in all

10 patients with sarcoidosis, the mediastinal nodes were visualized with FDG with a relatively high intensity (standard uptake value [SUV]=5.0), whereas FMT-PET demonstrated no or minimal uptake (SUV=0.8) at these sites. In contrast, in lung cancer, FMT and FDG demonstrated increased uptake. Therefore, this approach may be of value for distinguishing malignancy from sarcoidosis. PET may also provide some prognostic value in patients with sarcoidosis.

Overall, these data indicate that FDG as a single tracer is superior to the other existing agents for managing patients with sarcoidosis. Therefore, FDG-PET as a single modality seems to be quite promising for the detection and follow-up of disease activity in sarcoidosis. Well-designed prospective clinical studies are necessary to enhance its role in this disease, however.

Cardiac sarcoidosis

Cardiac sarcoidosis can be a benign and incidentally discovered condition; however, it can also be a life-threatening disorder because of its location and the extent of the granulomatous process. Clinical evidence of myocardial involvement is present in approximately 5% of patients with sarcoidosis, although autopsy studies indicate that subclinical cardiac involvement is present in a larger segment of this population.

The clinical manifestations of cardiac sarcoidosis are largely nonspecific. Myocardial involvement is common in patients with sarcoidosis who have cardiac symptoms and is unusual in those without such symptoms. For definitive diagnosis, an endomyocardial biopsy may be required, which is an established diagnostic procedure. Sampling error may produce false-negative results, however, because myocardial involvement may be nonuniform.

Chest radiography may reveal nonspecific findings, such as mild to moderate cardiomegaly, congestive heart failure, pericardial effusion, or a left ventricular aneurysm. The findings could be seen in combination with or without pulmonary sarcoidosis at various stages. Cardiac MRI is a new and exciting modality for this purpose, but experience for the diagnosis and monitoring of myocardial sarcoidosis is still limited. A variety of findings have been noted, including localized cardiac scarring and high-intensity areas on T1- and/or T2-weighted images. Gadolinium–diethylenetriamine penta-acetate (DTPA) enhancement permits early detection of cardiac involvement and assessment of the efficacy of steroid therapy [63–65]. In one series, late myocardial enhancement after gadolinium infusion, primarily involving the basal and lateral segments of the heart, was present in 19 patients, 8 of whom had normal exercise or Persantine thallium myocardial perfusion imaging [66]. The role of cardiac catheterization and coronary angiography is limited, but thrombosis, aneurysm formation, and partial or complete narrowing of the epicardial coronary arteries attributable to sarcoidosis can be visualized with the technique.

Conventional cardiac nuclear medicine procedures, such as Tl-201 and Tc-99m–labeled myocardial perfusion scans, may be helpful in patients with suspected cardiac sarcoidosis so as to determine myocardial or coronary artery involvement. For those patients who have known systemic sarcoidosis, perfusion defects strongly suggest cardiac involvement if atherosclerotic coronary disease is excluded as the underlying cause of these abnormalities. Decreased perfusion in the ventricular wall usually corresponds to the areas of fibrogranulomatous tissue replacement.

A thallium perfusion study is useful for monitoring the response to treatment in patients with myocardial sarcoidosis [67]. Okayama and coworkers [68] have proposed using a combination of cardiac perfusion and Ga-67 imaging to diagnose and monitor cardiac sarcoidosis. The authors believe that this combination may improve our ability to detect cardiac sarcoidosis. In this study, half of the patients with abnormal perfusion showed increased Ga-67 uptake. This report suggests that gallium-positive lesions may respond to corticosteroid treatment and thus improve myocardial function.

The role of 18F-FDG imaging in cardiac sarcoidosis is unclear at this time. A case report describes the usefulness of PET in the detection of cardiac sarcoidosis [69]. Another group studied the pattern of FDG uptake in patients with known cardiac sarcoidosis [70]. They concluded that focal uptake is a typical feature in this setting. This study also reported a crude comparison between FDG-PET and other nuclear medicine studies, such as Ga-67 and Tc-99m methoxy-isobutyl-isonitrile (MIBI) scans. The results showed that FDG-PET can detect cardiac sarcoidosis in cases in which Ga-67 or Tc-99m–MIBI scintigraphy seems negative. Another study showed that fasting FDG-PET can detect early inflammation caused by cardiac sarcoidosis even before the development of advanced fibrosis [71]. The combination of MRI and PET may improve the ability to obtain the required information for optimal management of these patients [72].

In a recent report, Yamagishi and coworkers [38] used N13-NH3 and F18-FDG-PET in assessing disease activity. They demonstrated equivalent sensitivity for both tests, but FDG seemed to be superior for monitoring treatment response and may be advantageous compared with conventional nuclear studies, such as Tl-201 and Ga-67, in this setting. False-negative results have been noted with this technique, however [73]. A patient with known active cardiac sarcoid and structural changes demonstrated by other tests failed to show abnormal activity on a Ga-67 or PET scan. Therefore, further research is needed to define the role of PET in cardiac sarcoidosis.

Neurosarcoidosis

Neurologic complications occur in approximately 5% of patients with sarcoidosis [74]. Neurosarcoidosis is a diagnostic dilemma in patients with known sarcoidosis who develop neurologic complaints and in patients presenting de novo with a constellation of findings consistent with the disease. Approximately 50% of patients with an eventual diagnosis of neurosarcoidosis present with neurologic difficulties at the time of initial diagnosis of the disease. One third of those with neurosarcoidosis develop more than one neurologic manifestation of the disease.

The imaging procedure of choice for the diagnosis of central nervous system (CNS) sarcoidosis is contrast-enhanced MRI. Meningeal or parenchymal enhancement suggests active inflammation with disruption of the blood-brain barrier with or without mass effects and hydrocephalus. Involvement of the optic nerve or other cranial nerves can be documented, and inflammation of the spinal cord and cauda equina is well seen on targeted anatomic images.

If the diagnosis remains in doubt, a meningeal, brain, or spinal cord biopsy is occasionally indicated. Performing a biopsy to establish the diagnosis rather than initiating empiric therapy should be considered if there is no evidence of systemic disease. A muscle and peripheral nerve biopsy can be easily performed if clinically warranted.

Reports related to the role of nuclear medicine procedures in neurosarcoidosis are scarce in the literature. There is a suggestion by one author [75] that FDG-PET might be helpful in overcoming some of the limitation of MRI. Other case reports of neurosarcoidosis [32,36,76] describe certain findings related to this disorder that reveal incidental findings using this technique. In general, PET is helpful for detecting clinically silent sites and for directing a biopsy to the appropriate site anywhere in the body for definitive diagnosis [74].

Other organs

As described earlier, sarcoidosis is a systemic disease and could involve any organ and/or system. Musculoskeletal system involvement is seen in up to 10% of affected patients [77]. Plain radiographs and MRI are the two main modalities commonly used for the diagnosis of musculoskeletal sarcoidosis, but the findings are nonspecific. There are case reports that describe FDG uptake in the muscle and bone sarcoidosis [35,37,78]. Other authors have described PET findings in cervical lymph node sarcoidosis [31] and skin lesions [24].

Summary

PET seems to be useful in the management of patients with sarcoidosis. Whole-body imaging with PET allows the detection of clinically silent sites or unsuspected lesions. FDG-PET is particularly useful for monitoring the response to treatment and demonstrates such effects in advance of those noted with anatomic techniques. Prospective well-designed research studies are required to determine the further role of this powerful modality in the management of this relatively common disorder.

References

[1] Hutchinson J. Case of livid papillary psoriasis. In: Illustrations of clinical surgery. London: J&A Churchill; 1877. p. 42.

[2] Muller-Quernheim J. Sarcoidosis: immunopathogenetic concepts and their clinical application. Eur Respir J 1998;12:716–38.

[3] Rybicki BA, Major M, Popovich Jr J, et al. Racial differences in sarcoidosis incidence: a 5-year study in a health maintenance organization. Am J Epidemiol 1997;145:234–41.

[4] Revsbech P. Is sarcoidosis related to exposure to pets or the housing conditions? A case-referent study. Sarcoidosis 1992;9:101–3.

[5] Baughman RP, Shipley R, Eisentrout CE. Predictive value of gallium scan, angiotensin-converting enzyme level, and bronchoalveolar lavage in two-year follow-up of pulmonary sarcoidosis. Lung 1987;165:371–7.

[6] Line BR, Hunninghake GW, Keogh BA, et al. Gallium-67 scanning to stage the alveolitis of sarcoidosis: correlation with clinical studies, pulmonary function studies, and bronchoalveolar lavage. Am Rev Respir Dis 1981;123:440–6.

[7] Beaumont D, Herry JY, Sapene M, et al. Gallium-67 in the evaluation of sarcoidosis: correlations with serum angiotensin-converting enzyme and bronchoalveolar lavage. Thorax 1982;37:11–8.

[8] Schoenberger CI, Line BR, Keogh BA, et al. Lung inflammation in sarcoidosis: comparison of serum angiotensin-converting enzyme levels with bronchoalveolar lavage and gallium-67 scanning assessment of the T lymphocyte alveolitis. Thorax 1982;37:19–25.

[9] Braude AC, Chamberlain DW, Rebuck AS. Pulmonary disposition of gallium-67 in humans: concise communication. J Nucl Med 1982;23:574–6.

[10] Braude AC, Cohen R, Rahmani R, et al. An in vitro gallium-67 lung index for the evaluation of sarcoidosis. Am Rev Respir Dis 1984;130:783–5.

[11] Tada A. [67-Gallium whole body scintigraphy and single photon emission computed tomography (SPECT) in sarcoidosis]. Nippon Rinsho 2002;60:1753–8 [in Japanese].

[12] Schuster DM, Alazraki N. Gallium and other agents in diseases of the lung. Semin Nucl Med 2002;32:193–211.

[13] Shorr AF, Helman DL, Lettieri CJ, et al. Depreotide scanning in sarcoidosis: a pilot study. Chest 2004;126:1337–43.

[14] Lebtahi R, Crestani B, Belmatoug N, et al. Somatostatin receptor scintigraphy and gallium scintigraphy in patients with sarcoidosis. J Nucl Med 2001;42:21–6.

[15] Alavi A, Gupta N, Alberini JL, et al. Positron emission tomography imaging in nonmalignant thoracic disorders. Semin Nucl Med 2002;32:293–321.

[16] El-Haddad G, Zhuang H, Gupta N, et al. Evolving role of positron emission tomography in the management of patients with inflammatory and other benign disorders. Semin Nucl Med 2004;34:313–29.

[17] Zhuang H, Alavi A. 18-Fluorodeoxyglucose positron emission tomographic imaging in the detection and monitoring of infection and inflammation. Semin Nucl Med 2002;32:47–59.

[18] Zhuang H, Yu JQ, Alavi A. Applications of fluorodeoxyglucose-PET imaging in the detection of infection and inflammation and other benign disorders. Radiol Clin North Am 2005;43:121–34.

[19] Yu JQ, Kung JW, Potenta S, et al. Chronic cholecystitis detected by FDG-PET. Clin Nucl Med 2004;29:496–7.

[20] Yu JQ, Zhuang H, Xiu Y, et al. Demonstration of increased FDG activity in Rosai-Dorfman disease on positron emission tomography. Clin Nucl Med 2004;29:209–10.

[21] Yu JQ, Kumar R, Xiu Y, et al. Diffuse FDG uptake in the lungs in aspiration pneumonia on positron emission tomographic imaging. Clin Nucl Med 2004;29:567–8.

[22] Kung J, Zhuang H, Yu JQ, et al. Intense fluorodeoxyglucose activity in pulmonary amyloid lesions on positron emission tomography. Clin Nucl Med 2003;28:975–6.

[23] Hughes JM, Rhodes CG, Brudin LH, et al. Contribution of the positron camera to studies of regional lung structure and function. Eur J Nucl Med 1987;13(Suppl):S37–41.

[24] Lewis PJ, Salama A. Uptake of fluorine-18-fluorodeoxyglucose in sarcoidosis. J Nucl Med 1994;35:1647–9.

[25] Alavi A, Buchpiguel CA, Loessner A. Is there a role for FDG PET imaging in the management of patients with sarcoidosis? J Nucl Med 1994;35:1650–2.

[26] Larson SM. Cancer or inflammation? A Holy Grail for nuclear medicine. J Nucl Med 1994;35:1653–5.

[27] Yasuda S, Shohtsu A, Ide M, et al. High fluorine-18

labeled deoxyglucose uptake in sarcoidosis. Clin Nucl Med 1996;21:983–4.

[28] Muggia FM, Conti PS. Seminoma and sarcoidosis: a cause for false positive mediastinal uptake in PET? Ann Oncol 1998;9:924.

[29] Kiatboonsri C, Resnick SC, Chan KM, et al. The detection of recurrent sarcoidosis by FDG-PET in a lung transplant recipient. West J Med 1998; 168:130–2.

[30] Gotway MB, Storto ML, Golden JA, et al. Incidental detection of thoracic sarcoidosis on whole-body 18-fluorine-2-fluoro-2-deoxy-D-glucose positron emission tomography. J Thorac Imaging 2000;15:201–4.

[31] Joe A, Hoegerle S, Moser E. Cervical lymph node sarcoidosis as a pitfall in F-18 FDG positron emission tomography. Clin Nucl Med 2001;26: 542–3.

[32] Xiu Y, Yu JQ, Cheng E, et al. Sarcoidosis demonstrated by FDG PET imaging with negative findings on gallium scintigraphy. Clin Nucl Med 2005;30:193–5.

[33] Brudin LH, Valind SO, Rhodes CG, et al. Fluorine-18 deoxyglucose uptake in sarcoidosis measured with positron emission tomography. Eur J Nucl Med 1994;21:297–305.

[34] Knopp MV, Bischoff HG. [Evaluation of pulmonary lesions with positron emission tomography]. Radiologe 1994;34:588–91 [in German].

[35] Kobayashi A, Shinozaki T, Shinjyo Y, et al. FDG PET in the clinical evaluation of sarcoidosis with bone lesions. Ann Nucl Med 2000;14:311–3.

[36] Dubey N, Miletich RS, Wasay M, et al. Role of fluorodeoxyglucose positron emission tomography in the diagnosis of neurosarcoidosis. J Neurol Sci 2002;205:77–81.

[37] Ludwig V, Fordice S, Lamar R, et al. Unsuspected skeletal sarcoidosis mimicking metastatic disease on FDG positron emission tomography and bone scintigraphy. Clin Nucl Med 2003;28:176–9.

[38] Yamagishi H, Shirai N, Takagi M, et al. Identification of cardiac sarcoidosis with (13)N-NH(3)/(18)F-FDG PET. J Nucl Med 2003;44:1030–6.

[39] Cook GJ, Fogelman I, Maisey MN. Normal physiological and benign pathological variants of 18-fluoro-2-deoxyglucose positron-emission tomography scanning: potential for error in interpretation. Semin Nucl Med 1996;26:308–14.

[40] Lodge MA, Lucas JD, Marsden PK, et al. PET study of 18FDG uptake in soft tissue masses. Eur J Nucl Med 1999;26:22–30.

[41] Zhuang H, Pourdehnad M, Lambright ES, et al. Dual time point 18F-FDG PET imaging for differentiating malignant from inflammatory processes. J Nucl Med 2001;42:1412–7.

[42] Kubota K, Itoh M, Ozaki K, et al. Advantage of delayed whole-body FDG-PET imaging for tumour detection. Eur J Nucl Med 2001;28:696–703.

[43] Aoki J, Watanabe H, Shinozaki T, et al. FDG-PET for preoperative differential diagnosis between benign and malignant soft tissue masses. Skeletal Radiol 2003;32:133–8.

[44] Aoki J, Watanabe H, Shinozaki T, et al. FDG PET of primary benign and malignant bone tumors: standardized uptake value in 52 lesions. Radiology 2001;219:774–7.

[45] Cremerius U, Wildberger JE, Borchers H, et al. Does positron emission tomography using 18-fluoro-2-deoxyglucose improve clinical staging of testicular cancer? Results of a study in 50 patients. Urology 1999;54:900–4.

[46] de Hemricourt E, De Boeck K, Hilte F, et al. Sarcoidosis and sarcoid-like reaction following Hodgkin's disease. Report of two cases. Mol Imaging Biol 2003;5:15–9.

[47] Grunwald F, Schomburg A, Bender H, et al. Fluorine-18 fluorodeoxyglucose positron emission tomography in the follow-up of differentiated thyroid cancer. Eur J Nucl Med 1996;23: 312–9.

[48] Higashi K, Ueda Y, Sakuma T, et al. Comparison of [(18)F]FDG PET and (201)Tl SPECT in evaluation of pulmonary nodules. J Nucl Med 2001;42: 1489–96.

[49] Kalff V, Hicks RJ, Ware RE, et al. The clinical impact of (18)F-FDG PET in patients with suspected or confirmed recurrence of colorectal cancer: a prospective study. J Nucl Med 2002;43: 492–9.

[50] Karapetis CS, Strickland AH, Yip D, et al. PET and PLAP in suspected testicular cancer relapse: beware sarcoidosis. Ann Oncol 2001;12:1485–8.

[51] Kubota K, Yamada S, Kondo T, et al. PET imaging of primary mediastinal tumours. Br J Cancer 1996;73:882–6.

[52] Nguyen AT, Akhurst T, Larson SM, et al. PET scanning with (18)F 2-fluoro-2-deoxy-D-glucose (FDG) in patients with melanoma. Benefits and limitations. Clin Positron Imaging 1999;2:93–8.

[53] Pitman AG, Hicks RJ, Kalff V, et al. Positron emission tomography in pulmonary masses where tissue diagnosis is unhelpful or not possible. Med J Aust 2001;175:303–7.

[54] Pitman AG, Hicks RJ, Binns DS, et al. Performance of sodium iodide based (18)F-fluorodeoxyglucose positron emission tomography in the characterization of indeterminate pulmonary nodules or masses. Br J Radiol 2002;75:114–21.

[55] van der Hoeven JJ, Krak NC, Hoekstra OS, et al. 18F-2-fluoro-2-deoxy-D-glucose positron emission tomography in staging of locally advanced breast cancer. J Clin Oncol 2004;22:1253–9.

[56] Maeda J, Ohta M, Hirabayashi H, et al. False positive accumulation in 18F fluorodeoxyglucose positron emission tomography scan due to sarcoid reaction following induction chemotherapy for lung cancer. Jpn J Thorac Cardiovasc Surg 2005;53:196–8.

[57] Yao M, Funk GF, Goldstein DP, et al. Benign lesions in cancer patients: case 1. Sarcoidosis after chemoradiation for head and neck cancer. J Clin Oncol 2005;23:640–1.

[58] Milman N, Mortensen J, Sloth C. Fluorodeoxyglucose PET scan in pulmonary sarcoidosis dur-

ing treatment with inhaled and oral corticosteroids. Respiration (Herrlisheim) 2003;70: 408–13.

[59] Hain SF, Beggs AD. C-11 methionine uptake in granulomatous disease. Clin Nucl Med 2004; 29:585–6.

[60] Halter G, Buck AK, Schirrmeister H, et al. [18F]3-deoxy-3′-fluorothymidine positron emission tomography: alternative or diagnostic adjunct to 2-[18F]-fluoro-2-deoxy-D-glucose positron emission tomography in the workup of suspicious central focal lesions? J Thorac Cardiovasc Surg 2004;127:1093–9.

[61] Yamada Y, Uchida Y, Tatsumi K, et al. Fluorine-18-fluorodeoxyglucose and carbon-11-methionine evaluation of lymphadenopathy in sarcoidosis. J Nucl Med 1998;39:1160–6.

[62] Oriuchi N, Inoue T, Tomiyoshi K. F-19-fluro-alpha-methyltyrosine (FMT) and F-18-flurodeoxyglucose (FDG) PET in patients with sarcoidosis. J Nucl Med 1999;40:878.

[63] Smedema JP, Truter R, de Klerk PA, et al. Cardiac sarcoidosis evaluated with gadolinium-enhanced magnetic resonance and contrast-enhanced 64-slice computed tomography. Int J Cardiol 2005.

[64] Smedema JP, Snoep G, van Kroonenburgh MP, et al. Cardiac involvement in patients with pulmonary sarcoidosis assessed at two university medical centers in the Netherlands. Chest 2005; 128:30–5.

[65] Smedema JP, Snoep G, van Kroonenburgh MP, et al. The additional value of gadolinium-enhanced MRI to standard assessment for cardiac involvement in patients with pulmonary sarcoidosis. Chest 2005;128:1629–37.

[66] Smedema JP, Snoep G, van Kroonenburgh MP, et al. Evaluation of the accuracy of gadolinium-enhanced cardiovascular magnetic resonance in the diagnosis of cardiac sarcoidosis. J Am Coll Cardiol 2005;45:1683–90.

[67] Mana J. Nuclear Imaging. 67 Gallium, 201 thallium, 18F-labeled fluoro-2-deoxy-D-glucose positron emission tomography. Clin Chest Med 1997; 18:799–811.

[68] Okayama K, Kurata C, Tawarahara K, et al. Diagnostic and prognostic value of myocardial scintigraphy with thallium-201 and gallium-67 in cardiac sarcoidosis. Chest 1995;107:330–4.

[69] Goto K, Okamoto E, Morita M, et al. [Cardiac sarcoidosis detected by FDG-PET]. Nippon Naika Gakkai Zasshi 2005;94:1396–8 [in Japanese].

[70] Ishimaru S, Tsujino I, Takei T, et al. Focal uptake on 18F-fluoro-2-deoxyglucose positron emission tomography images indicates cardiac involvement of sarcoidosis. Eur Heart J 2005;26: 1538–43.

[71] Okumura W, Iwasaki T, Toyama T, et al. Usefulness of fasting 18F-FDG PET in identification of cardiac sarcoidosis. J Nucl Med 2004;45: 1989–98.

[72] Smedema JP, van Erven L, Schreur JH, et al. [Cardiac sarcoidosis: improved prognosis through new diagnostic tests and treatment]. Ned Tijdschr Geneeskd 2005;149:1168–73 [in Dutch].

[73] Kaku B, Kanaya H, Horita Y, et al. Failure of follow-up gallium single-photon emission computed tomography and fluorine-18-fluorodeoxyglucose positron emission tomography to predict the deterioration of a patient with cardiac sarcoidosis. Circ J 2004;68:802–5.

[74] Stern BJ. Neurological complications of sarcoidosis. Curr Opin Neurol 2004;17:311–6.

[75] Braido F, Zolezzi A, Stea F, et al. Bilateral Gasser's ganglion sarcoidosis: diagnosis, treatment and unsolved questions. Sarcoidosis Vasc Diffuse Lung Dis 2005;22:75–7.

[76] Sponsler JL, Werz MA, Maciunas R, et al. Neurosarcoidosis presenting with simple partial seizures and solitary enhancing mass: case reports and review of the literature. Epilepsy Behav 2005; 6:623–30.

[77] Abril A, Cohen MD. Rheumatologic manifestations of sarcoidosis. Curr Opin Rheumatol 2004; 16:51–5.

[78] Aberg C, Ponzo F, Raphael B, et al. FDG positron emission tomography of bone involvement in sarcoidosis. AJR Am J Roentgenol 2004;182: 975–7.

POSITRON
EMISSION
TOMOGRAPHY

PET Clin 1 (2006) 153–162

Role of Fluorodeoxyglucose PET in Inflammatory Bowel Disease: A Review

Ewald Kresnik, MD[a],*, Peter Mikosch, MD[b],
Hans-Juergen Gallowitsch, MD[a], Susanne Kohlfürst, MD[a],
Isabell Igerc, MD[a], Peter Lind, MD[a]

- Pathophysiologic aspects and radiopharmaceutic agents for infection imaging
  Intact and fragment antibodies against granulocytes and labeled antibiotics
  Nonspecific human immunoglobulin
  White blood cell scintigraphy
  Fluorine-18 fluorodeoxyglucose PET for infection imaging
- Comparative studies with morphologic imaging
- Our results
- Summary
- References

Inflammatory bowel disease (IBD) is a term that is used for several inflammatory bowel disorders, such as colitis ulcerosa, Crohn's disease, and infectious colitis. IBD requires a complex diagnostic workup. Apart from the verification of IBD, it is also of clinical importance to assess the extent and activity of the disease and to detect associated complications so as to determine the most effective treatment.

Imaging methods like magnetic resonance colonography, ultrasonography, and endoscopy with biopsy are of diagnostic value. By applying scintigraphy, clinical questions regarding disease extent, activity, and associated complications in colitis can be answered with a single noninvasive investigation. Scintigraphy offers a complete survey of the whole intestinal tract, where the small and large

bowel intestinal tract can be seen. Conventional tracers like radiolabeled leukocytes and immunoscintigraphy with technetium-99m antigranulocyte antibodies are established and still widely used for the detection of inflammation. The importance of new imaging methods using fluorine-18 (F-18) fluorodeoxyglucose (FDG) in PET for detection of IBD is increasing.

Pathophysiologic aspects and radiopharmaceutic agents for infection imaging

Nuclear medicine provides information about pathophysiologic processes in the patient, whereas morphologic imaging methods provide information

[a] Department of Nuclear Medicine and Endocrinology, PET/CT Centre, General Hospital, St. Veiterstrasse 47, Klagenfurt A-9020, Austria
[b] Department of Internal Medicine and Gastroenterology, General Hospital, St. Veiterstrasse 47, Klagenfurt A-9020, Austria
* Corresponding author.
E-mail address: ewald.kresnik@lkh-klu.at (E. Kresnik).

doi:10.1016/j.cpet.2006.02.002

about morphologic changes occurring in a specific process. Host defense mechanisms in infections can be categorized as nonspecific or specific. Nonspecific imaging is directed against a wide range of infectious agents, whereas specific responses are directed against one particular microorganism [1,2].

Radiopharmaceutic agents and their uptake mechanism in inflammatory focus include the following:

1. Tc-99m intact and fragment granulocyte antibodies: specific uptake in the inflammatory focus. Granulocyte antibodies are directed against the nonspecific cross-reacting antigen 95 (NCA-95).
2. Tc-99m–labeled antibiotics: specific uptake by different microorganisms
3. Tc-99m/indium-111–labeled human immunoglobulin (HIG): nonspecific uptake in the inflammatory focus via increased capillary permeability
4. Tc-99m hexamethylpropyleneamine oxime (HMPAO)/In-111 oxine–labeled leukocytes: specific uptake in the inflammatory focus as a result of chemotactic activation
5. Fluorine-18 FDG-PET: uptake in inflammatory focus because of increased glucose metabolism

Intact and fragment antibodies against granulocytes and labeled antibiotics

The use of intact antibodies against granulocytes was first reported by Locher and colleagues [3]. The use of Tc-99m–labeled fragment antibodies NCA-95 Fab' (leukoscan) was reported by Becker and coworkers [4]. In a study comparing fragment antibody with the intact monoclonal antibody, the fragment antibody failed to detect the inflammatory bowel process in a patient with Crohn's disease, whereas the intact monoclonal antibody was able to detect the inflammation in that patient [5]. Similar results were reported by other authors. In their studies comparing white blood cell (WBC) scintigraphy with fragment antibodies, the leukoscan failed to detect inflammation in clinically active Crohn's disease, whereas WBC scintigraphy was able to identify the inflammatory process. Therefore, the leukoscan could not replace WBC scintigraphy in the investigation of IBD [6–8].

Some authors reported that Tc-99m–labeled antibiotics, which can be specifically metabolized by different microorganisms, may be indicative for septic inflammation but they provided false-negative results in patients with colitis ulcerosa [9,10]. Therefore, Tc-99m–labeled WBCs and intact granulocyte antibodies are preferred in case of abdominal infection or inflammation.

Another important aspect is the time of examination after tracer injection. For detection of in-

flammation using intact granulocyte antibodies in chronic inflammatory bowel disease (CIBD), 49% of segments could be detected at 2 hours after injection and 91% at 20 hours after injection [11]. In a prospective study of CIBD, Seggara and colleagues [12] found sensitivity, specificity, and accuracy rates of 61%, 100%, and 78% at 4 hours and rates of 79%, 92%, and 78% at 24 hours after injection, respectively. The activity increases in the bowel wall over the 24 hours after injection. This may be attributable to an antibody interaction with receptors on granulocytes within the bowel wall, with low fecal excretion [13]. Mahida and coworkers [14] also found low fecal excretion of 0.9% in patients with ulcerative colitis. The low excretion is most likely attributable to nonspecific Tc-99m excretion and not to CIBD. One explanation for increased tracer uptake in the bowel wall is cross-reactivity of NCA-95 antibodies with carcinoembryonic acid (CEA), which is elevated in 30% of patients with Crohn's disease or ulcerative colitis [15].

Nonspecific human immunoglobulin

Another tracer for infection imaging is nonspecific HIG. The usefulness of radiolabeled nonspecific HIG for the detection of intra-abdominal inflammation is reported, especially in patients with infections of the appendicular and periappendicular regions. A high sensitivity (100%) for radiolabeled nonspecific HIG could also be found in diverticulitis and diffuse colitis caused by *Escherichia coli* as well as in several patients with idiopathic ulcerative colitis [16].

White blood cell scintigraphy

WBC scintigraphy is widely used for infection imaging. The principal roles of leukocyte scanning in IBD are to establish the diagnosis, to identify disease segments to confirm relapse, to identify complications in Crohn's disease, and to quantify disease activity (especially when a new treatment is assessed).

Crohn's disease is associated with complications like fistulas and abscesses in 25% of patients. In case of an abscess, focally increased tracer uptake can be seen on a scan. Differentiation from physiologic bowel activity is possible because of the decreasing activity of the bowel over time, which is attributable to excretion into the bowel lumen and distal transit [17,18]. The sensitivity and specificity rates for the detection of purulent abscess are reported to be 90% to 95% and 93% to 100%, respectively [19,20]. Problems may occur in abscesses communicating with the bowel lumen. On late imaging scans, fistulas and sinuses can be suspected when there is no activity distal from a lesion or, occasionally, faint activity in the fistula can be seen [21,22]. Tracer activity in the bowel lumen has to be distinguished from mucosal bowel uptake. Nonspecific bowel activity can cause false-positive results [23–25]. Some authors have commented that nonspecific activity is faint and can be easily distinguished from mucosal uptake [26,27].

Scintigraphy with WBCs in CIBD enables localization of diseased bowel segments in the highly acute phase, with the danger of perforation during endoscopy, and in patients with stenosis, where endoscopy cannot pass the stenosis [28,29]. Scintigraphy with WBCs can also detect inflammatory activity in patients with minimal change colitis or early small bowel Crohn's disease, whereas radiologic or endoscopic investigations may often be normal or equivocal. Furthermore, in case of abnormal contrast bowel radiologic findings, differentiation is possible between inflammatory disease and lymphoid nodular hyperplasia [30,31].

In a comparison between WBC scintigraphy and a leukoscan for investigation of IBD, the leukoscan located inflammation, whereas WBC scintigraphy showed additional areas. The low sensitivity and specificity of the leukoscan preclude its use in the routine detection of infection, however [32]. The most common agent in adults used for WBC scintigraphy is Tc-99m HMPAO [33].The principal clinical indications include IBD, osteomyelitis, soft tissue sepsis, and occult fever. Tc-HMPAO has superior ability to identify small bowel involvement in patients with Crohn's disease reliably [28,34]. In a prospective survey of Crohn's disease, a 100% positive predictive value (PPV), 77% negative predictive value (NPV), sensitivity rate of 58%, and specificity rate of 100% were found. [35].

Another common agent for WBC scintigraphy is In-111. In-111–labeled leukocytes provide reliable images of the colon, but small bowel disease may be missed. This is attributable to a mobile small bowel as well as to rapid transit of its content [36]. It was also reported that different kinetic behaviors for In-111 oxine–labeled granulocytes may allow differentiation between diseased bowel segments and abdominal abscesses [12]. Soft abdominal infections can also be detected with labeled antibodies, however [16]. In a study using monoclonal antibodies for detection of inflammation, Lind and coworkers [37] found eight true-positive scans, two true-negative scans, and 1 false-negative scan.

Because of limitations of In-111–labeled leukocytes, however, the use of Tc-99m stannous colloid WBC scintigraphy for the evaluation of children with suspected IBD was assessed in a study by Paecock and colleagues [38]. The authors found a sensitivity of 88% and a specificity of 90% in IBD. The results are comparable to those of other WBC agents. Stannous colloid WBC scintigraphy should be preferred in children because of advantages in preparation and the smaller blood volume required [39].

In summary, for the detection of IBD in untreated patients, 80% to 98% sensitivity and 92% to 100% specificity can be found for scintigraphy [25,30,31, 40–43]. In contrast to the high specificity, there are also some reports on false-positive results attributable to mesenteric ischemia, carcinoma of the colon, or bleeding in the bowel [44–46].

Fluorine-18 fluorodeoxyglucose PET for infection imaging

Fluorine-18 FDG-PET has been shown to be useful in tumor diagnostics [47]. Malignant cells show enhanced glucose metabolism [48,49]. Increased FDG uptake in tumors is presumably the result of an increased number of glucose transporters in malignant cells. A comparable situation is also found in inflammation. Cytokines and growth factors increase the affinity of glucose transporters for deoxyglucose in inflammatory conditions, a mechanism that is absent in tumors [50–52].

Some authors reported positive results in FDG-PET attributable to abscess [53]. Furthermore, accumulation of F-18 FDG was found in peritumoral macrophages and granulation tissues [51]. A few studies tried to clarify the mechanism of F-18 FDG uptake in inflammatory cells in vitro, where mixed or pure preparations of WBCs were used [54–56]. It was thus legitimate to ask if F-18 FDG-PET was suitable for in vivo infection imaging. In a prospective study in patients with chronic osteomyelitis, Guhlmann and coworkers [57] showed a high sensitivity (100%) and specificity (92%) for PET. Also, noninfectious inflammation diseases like sarcoidosis show increased FDG uptake. The degree of FDG uptake is correlated with disease activity and can be used for monitoring response to treatment [58,59].

To date, only a few investigators have reported increased F-18 FDG uptake in acute enterocolitis [60–62]. The mechanism of tracer uptake is related to highly metabolic WBCs. Some reports have shown uptake in neutrophils and macrophages, because glycolysis is increased and hexose monophosphate shunt is more active [51,63].

Normal gut has patchy and unpredictable FDG uptake. Because of great turnover and shedding of intestinal mucosal cells into the bowel lumen, F-18 FDG uptake within mucosa may result in relevant intraluminal F-18 FDG concentrations. Bischof Delaloye and colleagues [64] calculated standard uptake values (SUVs) for normal intra-abdominal organs. The values were 2.58 ± 0.58 for spleen, 2.84 ± 1.06 for stomach, 2.95 ± 1.25 for gut, and 3.2 ± 0.79 for liver. The uptake in normal gut tends to be low and slightly lower than that of normal liver. On occasional instances, marked cecal uptake can be seen. The reason for this uptake is unknown and may be related to bacterial overgrowth.

The large intestine is a well-known site of physiologic uptake. In a study on 1068 healthy adults, Yasuda and coworkers [65] found 11% had FDG uptake in the intestine. Factors that influenced the uptake were gender (women showed more tracer uptake), age, and bowel condition (constipation). The reason why gender and age affect intestinal uptake is unknown. Constipation may be related to increased glucose metabolism in muscle movements, as documented for skeletal muscle exercise [66].

Stahl and colleagues [67] suggested that intestinal peristalsis attributable to smooth muscle activity may lead to accumulation of FDG in the intestinal tract. The authors could also demonstrate that FDG uptake is reduced after administration of N-butylscopolamin.

Kim and coworkers [68] also found intense colonic uptake with a focal pattern more frequently in patients with constipation, which is associated with increased muscular activity and results in high FDG uptake. Conversely, in five patients, Jadvar and colleagues [69] suggested that FDG uptake was not related to muscular peristalsis, because agents affecting the bowel motility, such as atropine and sincalide, did not influence FDG uptake. Mucosal uptake may be an alternative explanation.

Variants of FDG uptake in the bowel can also be caused by lymphoid tissue [70]. In a retrospective analysis of FDG colonic uptake, Tadlidil and coworkers [71] reported that a segmental pattern of FGD uptake was attributable to proctitis, infectious colitis, and lymphocytic and hemorrhagic colitis, whereas a nodular focal or multifocal pattern was found in polyps, adenoma, colon carcinoma, and mesenteric metastases. Diffuse intense uptake involving the whole colon had normal colonic finding. The grade of the uptake is variable, and it is not clear why proximal parts of the colon display higher levels and more variable patterns of FDG uptake than other colonic regions. It was suggested that a diffuse pattern with varying uptake level is more likely to be a physiologic variant than a pathologic process.

Diffusely increased colonic FDG uptake was reported in acute enterocolitis in a patient who was examined for colon carcinoma and in another patient with fever of unknown origin (FUO) [72, 73]. In their study, Lorenzen and colleagues [74] also found increased F-18 FDG uptake in the colon in 2 of 12 patients with FUO. One of these patients had *Yersinia* infection, and the other had tuberculous colitis. Fluorine-18 FDG uptake in acute colitis was also reported in a patient in whom there was no evidence of parasites or *Clostridium difficile* toxin [60].

In a case of pyrexia of unknown origin, Bleecker-Rovers and coworkers [75] found that the PPV for PET was 87% and the NPV was 95%. In patients with suspected focal infection or inflammation, the PPV and NPV were higher (95% and 100%, respectively). The results of PET were true positive in an abdominal abscess in two patients, Crohn's disease in one patient, and chronic granulomatous disease of the rectum in one patient. Physiologic bowel uptake led to false-positive results in one patient with fever and abdominal pain but normal morphological imaging, however. Conversely, the results of PET were false negative in one patient with Crohn's disease.

It is known that physiologic FDG uptake poses practical problem in the interpretation of PET images. It can lead to misinterpretation. Perhaps colonic lavage could help to reduce artifacts, because Miraldi and colleagues [76] reported on the elimination of artifactual accumulation with colonic lavage before examination in imaging of colorectal cancer.

Comparative studies with morphologic imaging

Morphologic imaging methods are well established and widely used for infection imaging. PET is a relatively new imaging method. The role of PET in infection imaging is gaining in importance.

In a comparative study of F-18 FDG-PET, hydro-MRI, and granulocyte scintigraphy with labeled antibodies for the detection of inflamed areas in the terminal ileum and colon of patients with Crohn's disease, Neurath and coworkers [77] found sensitivity rates of 85%, 67%, and 41%, respectively, and specificity of rates of 89%, 93%, and 100%, respectively. Hydro-MRI was insufficient for the detection of inflamed areas in the transverse descending colon and rectosigmoid.

FDG-PET seems to be a reliable noninvasive tool for simultaneous detection of inflamed areas in the small and large bowel. The "gold standard" for the diagnosis and monitoring of complications of Crohn's disease is endoscopy with consecutive histologic evaluation of biopsy specimens. FDG-PET detected mild inflamed areas in Crohn's disease that had been proven by histology; however, in endoscopy, the inflamed areas were normal [78,79].

Our results

In a preliminary study, F-18 FDG-PET was used to evaluate the usefulness of metabolic imaging in the early diagnosis of colitis [79]. Five women who had been diagnosed as having an early clinical stage of colitis were investigated. One patient suffered from *Salmonella* infection that showed increased tracer uptake in the entire colon. Two had collagenous colitis, with increased tracer uptake in the ascending colon in one and in the sigmoid and rectum in the other. Another two had eosinophilic colitis. PET showed an increased tracer uptake in the sigmoid in one and a transverse descending colon in the other. Morphologic imaging was not suspicious in the patients with collagenous and eosinophilic colitis. Colonoscopy did not show any abnormalities. Guided by positive PET findings, multiple biopsies were taken from the areas with increased tracer uptake. Histologic examination confirmed the diagnosis of collagenous and eosinophilic colitis [Fig. 1]. In patients with an early clinical stage of collagenous or eosinophilic colitis, morphologic imaging is usually nondiagnostic. In the present cases, the radiologic and endoscopic examinations also showed no abnormalities. PET was able to detect colitis at an early clinical stage when morphologic imaging was nondiagnostic. Fluorine-18 FDG-PET imaging in patients with possible colitis is encouraging.

Our results are in agreement with those of other authors, who have also reported that the advantages in comparing PET scintigraphy with conventional imaging are the high sensitivity in chronic low-grade infections, high target-to-background ratio, and early imaging [80–82].

Pio and colleagues [83] reported in their first study on the quantification of bowel inflammation using FDG-labeled WBCs that the intensity of foci measured in PET correlated well with histopathologic measurements of the degree of inflammation. The study was performed only in three human subjects, however. In the future, FDG labeling of WBCs might help to differentiate between FDG

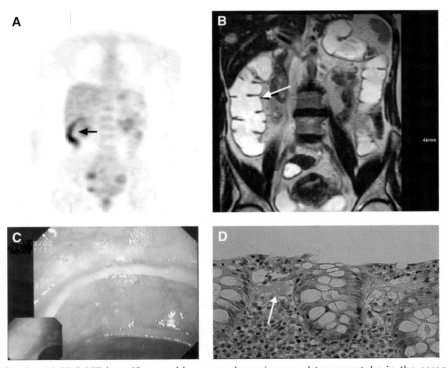

Fig. 1. (*A*) Fluorine-18 FDG-PET in a 48-year-old woman shows increased tracer uptake in the ascending colon (*arrow*). (*B*) Magnetic resonance colonography of the ascending colon also shows no abnormalities. (*C*) Colonoscopy shows no abnormalities. (*D*) Histologic section of the ascending colon demonstrates collagenous colitis with damage of the surface epithelial cells, an increased number of intraepithelial lymphocytes, and a thick subepithelial collagen band (*arrow*) (Masson's trichrome, original magnification ×200). (*From* Kresnik E, Gallowitsch HJ, Mikosch P, et al. 18F-FDG positron emission tomography in the early diagnosis of enterocolitis: preliminary results. Eur J Nucl Med 2002;29:1391; with permission of Springer Science and Business Media.)

uptake attributable to intestinal inflammation and that attributable to colorectal cancer. Another study reported on dual-point FDG-PET imaging for differentiating malignant from inflammatory processes [84]. The authors demonstrated that the SUV significantly increased in tumors over time, whereas the SUV of inflammatory lesions decreased over time. Ichiya and coworkers [85] reported in their study on FDG-PET in infectious lesions that the patterns of the time activity curves in acute or chronic active lesions showed an increase without an initial peak or plateau, whereas the healing lesions demonstrated an increase with an initial peak. In infectious lesions, FDG accumulated in migratory inflammatory cells, causative microorganisms, and granulation tissue [86]. It was postulated that migratory inflammatory cells, like neutrophils and microorganisms, play a role in the acute stage, whereas in granulation tissue, lymphocytes play a role in the healing stage. It is known that neutrophils use glucose as a source of energy. Glucose use in neutrophils is 10 times higher than that in lymphocytes. Acute active lesions showed higher FGD uptake than in chronic active lesions. Furthermore, microorganisms metabolize glucose as a source of energy. Therefore, it is possible that a portion of FDG administered is incorporated into causative microorganisms [87,88].

A disadvantage of fluorodeoxyglucose positron emission tomography imaging is the limited anatomic information that it provides. New imaging modalities like combined PET/CT may help to reduce false-positive results, because nonspecific tracer uptake within the colon can be distinguished from uptake in the bowel wall. In a study on the advantages of combined PET/CT in 265 patients, Igerc and coworkers [89] found that PET/CT provided additional information (eg, better delineation, tumor extent, topographic information) in 70.8% of cases. The results had an impact on the management of 14.3% of their patients. Also, in abdominal scintigraphy, anatomic detail provided by PET/CT imaging may help to avoid misinterpretation of tracer excretion into the bowel lumen. Nevertheless, interpretation of PET/CT images using oral contrast should be done with caution, because oral contrast can cause overestimation of tissue FDG concentration; therefore, artifacts with false-positive results may occur. Sun and colleagues [90] found that the average SUV of the ascending colon, transverse colon, and rectum in patients who had received oral contrast agent was significantly higher than that of patients in the control group. There were no significant differences in the average SUV of the stomach, jejunum, ileum, or descending colon. Negative oral contrast prevents artifacts in PET. In a study of 49 patients, Hausegger and colleagues [91] investigated the negative, vegetarian-based substance, oral contrast material (Mucofalk, Freiburg, Germany) in whole-body PET/CT. Distention of the small bowel was excellent or good in 85% of patients and poor in 15% of patients. Mild tracer uptake in the small bowel was observed in 4% of patients. Mucofalk did not interfere with image interpretation and can be used as a negative oral contrast medium in PET/CT studies. To date, however, only a few reports on the use of PET/CT have been published in the literature. These studies deal with oncologic questions. There is no study available on using PET/CT in inflammation. Future studies are necessary to elucidate the usefulness of coincident imaging.

Summary

Scintigraphy is a functional imaging method that offers a complete survey of the whole intestinal tract, where the small and the large bowel tract can be seen. Scintigraphy has an important role in the localization of diseased bowel segments in the highly acute phase when endoscopy is problematic because of stenosis or danger of perforation during endoscopy. Scintigraphy has high sensitivity and specificity for detection of complications in Crohn's disease, such as abscesses and fistulas. Fluorine-18 FDG-PET is a metabolic imaging method. PET has been shown to be useful for the detection of bowel inflammation at an early clinical stage when morphologic imaging was nondiagnostic. PET can also help to demonstrate inflammation in stenosis, which influences the therapeutic strategy in Crohn's disease. In case of FUO, metabolic imaging has been shown to be more specific than other modalities. New imaging modalities like combined PET/CT help to reduce false-positive results, because physiologic tracer uptake can be easily distinguished from pathologic lesions as a result of the anatomic detail provided by CT.

References

[1] Woods G, Gutierrez Y, Walker D, et al. Diagnostic pathology of infectious disease. Philadelphia: Lea & Febiger; 1993.

[2] Goldenberg DM, Sharkey RM, Udem S, et al. Immunoscintigraphy of Pneumocystis carinii pneumonia in AIDS patients. J Nucl Med 1994; 35:1028–34.

[3] Locher JT, Seybold K, Andres RY, et al. Imaging of inflammatory and infectious lesions after injection of radioiodinated monoclonal antigranulocyte antibodies. Nucl Med Commun 1986;7: 659–70.

[4] Becker W, Bair J, Behr T, et al. Detection of soft tissue infections and osteomyelitis using a technetium-99m-labeled antigranulocyte monoclonal antibody fragment. J Nucl Med 1994;35:1436–43.

[5] Kresnik E, Gallowitsch HJ, Mikosch P, et al. Immunoscintigraphy of an inflammatory bowel process in Crohn's disease with a technetium-99m-labelled fragment (MN3 Fab') and with an intact monoclonal anti-granulocyte antibody (Mab BW 250/183). Clin Nucl Med 1999;24:64–5.

[6] Kapsoritakis AN. 99m-Tc-leukoscan in the evaluation of inflammatory bowel disease. Eur J Nucl Med 2002;29:1098.

[7] Stokkel MPM, Reigman HIE, Pauwels EKJ. Scintigraphic head-to-head comparison between 99mTc-WBCs and 99mTc-leukoscan in the evaluation of inflammatory bowel disease: a pilot study. Eur J Nucl Med 2002;29:251–4.

[8] Kolkman JJ, Falke TH, Roos JC, et al. Computed tomography and granulocyte scintigraphy in active inflammatory bowel disease. Comparison with endoscopy operative findings. Dig Dis Sci 1996;41:641–50.

[9] Gallowitsch HJ, Heinisch M, Mikosch P, et al. Tc-99m ciprofloxacin in clinically selected patients suspected for peripheral osteomyelitis, spondylodiscitis and fever of unknown origin: preliminary results. Nuklearmedizin 2002;41:30–6.

[10] Bomanji J, Solanki KK, Britton KE, et al. Imaging infection with Tc-99m–radiolabelled "infecton". Eur J Nucl Med 1993;20:834.

[11] Becker W, Fleig W, Marienhagen J, et al. Diagnostische Bedeutung der intestinalen Aktivität bei der Immunszintigraphie mit Tc-99m-NCA-95-Antikörpern. Nuklearmedizin 1990;229:47–8.

[12] Seggara I, Roca M, Ballielas C, et al. Granulocyte-specific monoclonal antibody technetium-99m BW 250/183 and In-111-oxine labelled leukocyte scintigraphy in inflammatory bowel disease. Eur J Nucl Med 1991;18:715–9.

[13] Becker W, Goldenberg DM, Wolf F, et al. The use of monoclonal antibodies and antibody fragments in the imaging of infectious lesions. Semin Nucl Med 1994;24:1–13.

[14] Mahida YR, Perkins AC, Frier M, et al. Monoclonal granulocyte antibody in inflammatory bowel disease: a preliminary report. Nucl Med Commun 1992;13:330–5.

[15] Fischbach W, Mössner J, Seyschab H, et al. Tissue carcinoembryonic antigen and DNA aneuploidy in precancerous and cancerous colorectal lesions. Cancer 1990;65:1820–4.

[16] Serafini AN, Garty I, Vargas-Cuba R, et al. Clinical evaluation of a scintigraphic method for diagnosing inflammations/infections using indium-111-labeled nonspecific human IgG. J Nucl Med 1991;32:2227–32.

[17] Becker W, Fischbach W, Reiners C, et al. Three phase blood cell scan: diagnostic validity in abdominal inflammatory diseases. J Nucl Med 1986;27:1109–15.

[18] Weldon MJ, Joseph EA, Frech A, et al. Comparison of 99m Tc hexamethylpropylene-amine oxime labelled leukocyte with 111-indium tropolonate labelled granulocyte scanning and ultrasound in the diagnosis of intraabdominal abscess. Gut 1995;37:557–64.

[19] Wheeler JG, Slack NF, Duncan A, et al. The diagnosis of intra-abdominal abscesses in patients with severe Chiron's disease. Q J Med 1992;82:159–67.

[20] Saverymuttu SH, Maltby P, Batman P, et al. False positive localisation of indium-111 granulocytes in colonic carcinoma. Br J Radiol 1986;59:373–7.

[21] Spinellei F, Milella M, Sara R, et al. The 99mTc–HMPAO leukocyte scan: an alternative to radiology and endoscopy in evaluating the extent and the activity of inflammatory bowel disease. J Nucl Biol Med 1991;35:82–7.

[22] Even-Sapir E, Barnes DC, Martin RH, et al. Indium-111-white blood cell scintigraphy in Crohn's patients with fistulae and sinus tracts. J Nucl Med 1994;35:245–50.

[23] Gibson P, Lichtenstein M, Salehi N, et al. Value of positive technetium-99m leukocyte scans in predicting intestinal inflammations. Gut 1991;32:1502–7.

[24] Ivancevic V, Munz DL. Nonspecific bowel activity in 99mTc-labelled monoclonal anti-granulocyte antibody imaging. Nucl Med Commun 1992;13:899–900.

[25] Lantto E, Jarvi K, Krekela I, et al. Technetium-99m hexamethyl propylene amine oxine leukocytes in the assessment of disease activity in inflammatory bowel disease. Eur J Nucl Med 1992;19:14–8.

[26] Weldon MJ, Masoomi AM, Britten AJ, et al. Quantification of inflammatory bowel disease activity using technetium-99m HMPAO labelled leukocyte single photon emission computerized tomography (SPECT). Gut 1995;36:243–50.

[27] Allan RA, Sladen GE, Bassingham S, et al. Comparison of simultaneous 99mTc-HMPAO and 111In oxine labelled white cell scans in the assessment of inflammatory bowel disease. Eur J Nucl Med 1993;20:195–200.

[28] Arndt JW, Van der Sluys Veer A, Block D, et al. Prospective comparative study of Tc-99m-WBCs and indium-111 granulocytes for the examination of inflammatory bowel disease. J Nucl Med 1993;34:1052–7.

[29] Allan RA, Sladen GE, Bassingham S, et al. Comparison of simultaneous Tc-99m-HMPAO and indium-111-oxine labelled white blood cell scans in the assessment of inflammatory bowel disease. Eur J Nucl Med 1993;20:195–200.

[30] Saverymuttu SH, Peters AM, Crofton ME, et al. 111-Indium autologous granulocytes in the detection of inflammatory bowel disease. Gut 1985;26:955–60.

[31] Charron M, Del Rosario F, Kocoshis S. Assessment of terminal ileal and colonic inflammation in Crohn's disease with 99m-Tc-WBC. Acta Pediatr 1999;88:193–8.

[32] Kerry JE, Marshall C, Griffiths PA, et al. Comparison between Tc-HMPAO labelled white cells and Tc leukoscan in the investigation of inflammatory bowel disease. Nucl Med Commun 2005;26: 245–51.

[33] Peters AM, Danpure HJ, Osman S, et al. Clinical experience with 99m-Tc-hexamethylpropyleneamineoxime for labeling leukocytes and imaging inflammation. Lancet 1986;2:946–9.

[34] Scholmerich J, Schmidt E, Shumichen C, et al. Scintigraphic assessment of bowel involvement and disease activity in Crohn's disease using Tc-99m hexamethylpropyleneamine oxime as a leukocyte label. Gastroenterology 1998;95: 1287–93.

[35] Lachter J, Isserof HN, Yasin K, et al. Radiolabeled leukocyte imaging in inflammatory bowel disease: a prospective blinded evaluation. Hepatogastroenterology 2003;53:1439–41.

[36] Saverymuttu SH, Peters AM, Hodgson HJ, et al. Indium-111 leukocyte scanning: comparison with radiology for imaging of colon in inflammatory bowel disease. BMJ 1982;285:255–7.

[37] Lind P, Langsteger W, Költringer P, et al. Immunoscintigraphy of inflammatory processes with a technetium-99m labelled monoclonal antibody (Mab BW 250/183). J Nucl Med 1990;31: 417–23.

[38] Paecock K, Porn U, Howman-Giles R, et al. 99m Tc-stannous colloid white cell scintigraphy in childhood inflammatory bowel disease. J Nucl Med 2004;45:261–5.

[39] Hughes DK. Nuclear medicine and infection detection: the relative effectiveness of imaging with 111In-oxine-, 99mTc-HMPAO-, and 99mTc-stannous fluoride colloid-labeled leukocytes and with 67Ga-citrate. J Nucl Med Technol 2003;31: 196–201.

[40] Del Rosario MA, Fitzgerald JF, Siddiqui AR, et al. Clinical applications of Tc-99m hexamethyl propylene amine oxime leukocyte scan in children with inflammatory bowel disease. J Pediatr Gastroenterol Nutr 1999;28:63–70.

[41] Guimbaud R, Beades E, Chauvelot-Moachon L, et al. Technetium 99m hexamethyl propylene amine oxime leukocyte scintigraphy in patients with ulcerative colitis : correlation with clinical, biologic, endoscopic, and pathologic intensity, and local release of interleukin 8. Gastrointest Endosoc 1998;48:491–6.

[42] Barabino A, Gattorno M, Cabria M, et al. 99mTc-white cell scanning to detect gut inflammation in children with inflammatory bowel disease or spondyloarthropathies. Clin Exp Rheumatol 1998;16:327–34.

[43] Sciarretta G, Furno A, Mazzoni M, et al. Technetium-99m hexamethyl propylene amine oxime granulocyte scintigraphy in Crohn's disease: diagnostic and clinical relevance. Gut 1993; 34:1364–9.

[44] Wheeler JG, Baker AJ, Slack NF. Case report: extensive uptake of 99mTc-HMPAO labelled leukocytes in the small bowel of patient with mesenteric ischemia. Clin Radiol 1998;53: 227–8.

[45] Fisher MF, Rudd TG. In-111-labeled leukocyte imaging: false positive study due to acute gastrointestinal bleeding. J Nucl Med 1983;24:803–4.

[46] Saverymuttu SH, Crofton ME, Peters AM, et al. Indium-111 tropolonate leukocyte scanning in the detection of intra-abdominal abscesses. Clin Radiol 1983;34:593–6.

[47] Reske S, Bares R, Büll U, et al. Klinische Wertigkeit der Positronenemissionstomographie (PET) bei onkologischen Fragestellungen: Ergebnisse einer interdisziplinären Konsensuskonferenz. Nuklearmedizin 1996;35:42–52.

[48] Mac Keehan WL. Glycolysis, glutaminolysis and cell proliferation. Cell Biol Int 1982;6:635–50.

[49] Weber G. Enzymology of cancer cells. N Engl J Med 1977;296:541–51.

[50] Zhuang H, Alavi A. 18-fluorodeoxyglucose positron emission tomographic imaging in the detection and monitoring of infection and inflammation. Semin Nucl Med 2002;32:47–59.

[51] Alavi A, Zhuang H. Finding infection-help from PET. Lancet 2001;38:1386.

[52] Paik JY, Lee CH, Choe YS, et al. Augmented 18F-FDG uptake in activated monocytes occurs during the priming process and involves tyrosine kinases and protein kinase. J Nucl Med 2004;45: 124–8.

[53] Sasaki M, Ichiya Y, Kuwabara Y, et al. Ringlike uptake of F-18- FDG in brain abscess: a PET study. J Comput Assist Tomogr 1990;14:486–7.

[54] Osman S, Danpure HJ. The use of 2-(18) fluoro-2-deoxy-d-glucose as a potential in vitro agent for labeling human granulocytes for clinical studies by positron emission tomography. J Radiat Appl Instrum 1992;19:183–90.

[55] Forstrom LA, Mullan BP, Hung JC, et al. 18F-FDG labelling of human leukocytes. Nucl Med Commun 2000;21:691–4.

[56] Becker W, Meller J. The role of nuclear medicine in infection and inflammation. Lancet Infect Dis 2001;1:326–33.

[57] Guhlmann A, Brech-Krauss D, Suger G, et al. Chronic osteomyelitis: detection with FDG PET and correlative histopathologic findings. Radiology 1998;206:749–54.

[58] Brudin LH, Valind SO, Rhodes CG, et al. Fluorine-18 deoxyglucose uptake in sarcoidosis measured with positron emission tomography. Eur J Nucl Med 1994;21:297–305.

[59] Love C, Tomas MB, Tronco GG, et al. FDG PET of infection and inflammation. Radiographics 2005;25:1357–68.

[60] Meyer MA. Diffusely increased colonic F-18 FDG uptake in acute enterocolitis. Clin Nucl Med 1995; 20:434–5.

[61] Hannah A, Scott AM, Akhurst T, et al. Abnormal colonic accumulation of fluorine-18-FDG in pseudomembranous colitis. J Nucl Med 1996;37:1683–5.

[62] Kresnik E, Mikosch P, Gallowitsch HJ, et al. F-18 fluorodeoxyglucose positron emission tomography in the diagnosis of inflammatory bowel disease. Clin Nucl Med 2001;26:867.

[63] Larson SM. Cancer or inflammation? A holy grail for nuclear medicine [editorial]. J Nucl Med 1994;35:1653–5.

[64] Bischof Delaloye A, Wahl RL. How high level of FDG abdominal activity is considered normal? [abstract]. J Nucl Med 1995;36(Suppl):106P.

[65] Yasuda S, Takahashi W, Takagi S, et al. Factors influencing physiological FDG uptake in the intestine. Tokaj J Exp Clin Med 1998;23:241–4.

[66] Kostakoglu L, Wong JCH, Barrington SF, et al. Speech-related visualization of laryngeal muscles with fluorine-18-FDG. J Nucl Med 1996;37:1771–3.

[67] Stahl A, Weber WA, Avril N, et al. Effect of N-butyl-scopolamine on intestinal uptake of fluorine-18-fluorodeoxyglucose in PET imaging of the abdomen. Nuklearmedizin 2000;39:214–45.

[68] Kim S, Chung JK, Kim BT, et al. Relationship between gastrointestinal F-18-fluorodeoxyglucose accumulation and gastrointestinal symptoms in whole-body PET. Clin Positron Imaging 1999;2:273–80.

[69] Jadvar H, Schambye RB, Segall GM. Effect of atropine and sincalide on the intestinal uptake of F-18 fluorodeoxyglucose. Clin Nucl Med 1999;24:965–7.

[70] Cook GJR, Fogelman I, Maisey MN. Normal physiological and benign pathological variants of 18-fluoro-deoxyglucose positron emission tomography scanning: potential for error in interpretation. Semin Nucl Med 1996;26:308–14.

[71] Tadlidil R, Jadvar H, Badin JR, et al. Incidental colonic fluorodeoxyglucose uptake: correlation with colonoscopic and histopathologic findings. Radiology 2002;224:783–7.

[72] Meyer MA. Diffusely increased colonic F-18 FDG uptake in acute enterocolitis. Clin Nucl Med 1995;20:434–5.

[73] Ruf J, Griebenow B, Stiller B, et al. Detection of infectious colitis by 18F-fluorodeoxyglucose-positron emission tomography in a child receiving intensive care after surgery. Pediatr Radiol 2005;35:702–5.

[74] Lorenzen J, Buchert R, Bohuslavizki KH. Value of FGDG PET in patients with fever of unknown origin. Nucl Med Commun 2001;22:779–83.

[75] Bleecker-Rovers CP, Kleijn E, Corstens FHM, et al. Clinical value of FDG PET in patients with fever of unknown origin and patients suspected of focal infection or inflammation. Eur J Nucl Med Mol Imaging 2004;31:29–37.

[76] Miraldi F, Vesselle H, Faulhaber PF, et al. Elimination of artifactual accumulation of FDG in PET imaging of colorectal cancer. Clin Nucl Med 1998;23:3–7.

[77] Neurath MF, Schunk V, Holtmann M, et al. Noninvasive assessment of Crohn's disease activity: a comparison of 18F-fluorodeoxyglucose positron emission tomography, hydromagnetic resonance imaging, and granulocyte scintigraphy with labeled antibodies. Am J Gastroenterol 2002;97:1978–85.

[78] Bicik I, Bauerfeind P, Breitenbach T, et al. Inflammatory bowel disease activity measured by positron-emission tomography. Lancet 1997;350:262.

[79] Kresnik E, Gallowitsch HJ, Mikosch P, et al. 18F-FDG positron emission tomography in the early diagnosis of enterocolitis: preliminary results. Eur J Nucl Med 2002;29:1389–92.

[80] De Winter F, van de Wiele C, Vogelaers D, et al. Fluorine-18 fluorodeoxyglucose-positron emission tomography: a highly accurate imaging modality for the diagnosis of chronic musculoskeletal infections. J Bone Joint Surg Am 2001;83:651–60.

[81] Sugawara Y, Braun DK, Kison PV, et al. Rapid detection of human infections with fluorine 18 fluorodeoxyglucose and positron emission tomography: preliminary results. Eur J Nucl Med 1998;25:1238–43.

[82] Sugawara Y, Gutowsky TD, Fisher SJ, et al. Uptake of positron emission tomography tracers in experimental bacterial infections: a comparative biodistribution study of radiolabeled FDG, thymidine, L-methionine, 67Ga-citrate, and 125I-HSA. Eur J Nucl Med 1996;26:333–41.

[83] Pio BS, Byrne FR, Aranda R, et al. Noninvasive quantification of bowel inflammation through positron emission tomography imaging of 2-deoxy-2-(18F)fluoro-D-glucose-labeled white blood cells. Mol Imaging Biol 2003;5:271–7.

[84] Zhuang H, Pourdehnad M, Lambright ES, et al. Dual time point 18F-FDG PET imaging for differentiating malignant from inflammatory process. J Nucl Med 2001;42:1412–7.

[85] Ichiya Y, Kuwabaka Y, Sasaki M, et al. FDG-PET in infectious lesions: The detection and assessment of lesion activity. Ann Nucl Med 1996;10:185–91.

[86] Daley JM, Shearer JD, Mastrofrancesco B, et al. Glucose metabolism in injured tissue. A longitudinal study. Surgery 1990;107:187–92.

[87] West J, Morton DJ, Esmann V, et al. Carbohydrate metabolism in leukocytes. Metabolic activities of the macrophage. Arch Biochem Biophys 1968;124:85–90.

[88] Anderson RL, Wood WA. Carbohydrate metabolism in microorganisms. Annu Rev Microbiol 1969;23:539–78.

[89] Igerc I, Gallowitsch HJ, Kohlfürst S, et al. The incremental value of combined 18F-fluorodeoxy-

glucose (FDG)-PET/contrast enhanced computed tomography (ceCT) in oncology patients in reducing false positive results [abstract]. Eur J Nucl Med 2005;32(Suppl):S154.

[90] Sun XG, Xiu LR, Wan LR, et al. Oral contrast agent during PET/CT scan could increase FDG uptake in colon and rectum [abstract]. Eur J Nucl Med 2005;32(Suppl):S80.

[91] Hausegger K, Reinprecht P, Kau T, et al. Clinical experience with a commercially available negative oral contrast medium in PET/CT. Fortschr Rontgenstr 2005;177:796–9.

POSITRON
EMISSION
TOMOGRAPHY

PET Clin 1 (2006) 163–177

Value of 18-Fluoro-2-Deoxyglucose PET in the Management of Patients with Fever of Unknown Origin

Ghassan El-Haddad, MD[a], Abass Alavi, MD[a],
Hongming Zhuang, MD, PhD[a,b],*

- Differential diagnosis
  - *Infections*
  - *Malignancies*
  - *Noninfectious inflammatory diseases*
  - *Miscellaneous*
- Evaluation of the patient with fever of unknown origin by conventional methods
  - *Radiographic evaluation*
  - *General nuclear medicine*
- 18-Fluoro-2-deoxyglucose PET
  - *Mechanism of action*
  - *Basis for the use of 18-fluoro-2-deoxyglucose PET in fever of unknown origin*
- *18-Fluoro-2-deoxyglucose PET versus other nuclear medicine techniques*
- *18-Fluoro-2-deoxyglucose PET versus anatomic imaging*
- *Limitations of 18-fluoro-2-deoxyglucose PET*
- *18-Fluoro-2-deoxyglucose PET and fever of unknown origin in the literature*
- Summary
- References

Most febrile illnesses resolve before a diagnosis is made, or characteristic symptoms and signs develop that lead to the correct diagnosis. Fever of unknown origin (FUO) is reserved for patients with a prolonged febrile illness without an established cause in spite of an intense search to identify the source. Despite the fact that most FUOs are self-limited, they pose a major challenge to the attending physicians and supportive staff. Certain diseases that are not recognized promptly and treated appropriately can cause significant morbidity or even mortality in this population.

The definition of FUO as set forth in 1961 by Petersdorf and Beeson [1] after a prospective analysis of 100 cases was (1) a temperature of greater than 38.3°C (101°F) on several occasions, (2) a duration of more than 3 weeks, and (3) failure to reach a diagnosis despite 1 week of inpatient investigation. This definition has since been revised, and as such, there is a heavy emphasis on the ambulatory evaluation of these patients. Currently, there are four categories of FUO: classic, nosocomial, immune deficient (neutropenic), and HIV related [2,3]. The four subcategories of the differen-

a Department of Radiology, University of Pennsylvania School of Medicine, Hospital of the University of Pennsylvania, Philadelphia, PA 19104, USA
b Department of Radiology, The Children's Hospital of Philadelphia, 34th Street and Civic Center Boulevard, Philadelphia, 110 Donner Building, 3400 Spruce Street, PA 19104, USA
* Corresponding author. Department of Radiology, The Children's Hospital of Philadelphia, 34th Street and Civic Center Boulevard, Philadelphia, PA 19104.
E-mail address: zhuang@email.chop.edu (H. Zhuang).

1556-8598/06/$ – see front matter © 2006 Elsevier Inc. All rights reserved.
doi:10.1016/j.cpet.2006.01.003
pet.theclinics.com

tial diagnosis of FUO are infections, malignancies, autoimmune conditions, and miscellaneous.

Classic FUO is a fever that is higher than 38.3°C on several occasions of at least 3 weeks' duration and an uncertain diagnosis after 3 days of hospitalization, three outpatient visits, or 1 week of "intelligent and invasive" ambulatory investigation [2,4]. Classic FUO is close to the earlier definition of FUO but is somewhat broader, differing only with regard to the prior requirement for 1 week's study in the hospital. The most common causes of classic FUO are infection, malignancy, collagen vascular disease, and drug fever.

Nosocomial FUO refers to a temperature of 38.3°C (101°F) or greater on several occasions in a hospitalized patient who is receiving acute care and in whom infection was not manifest or incubating on admission. The diagnosis is made after 3 days of illness under exploration, including at least 2 days' incubation of cultures. Common etiologies of nosocomial FUO are *Clostridium difficile* enterocolitis, septic thrombophlebitis, pulmonary embolism, and drug-induced fever. In patients with nasogastric tubes, sinusitis may be a cause of nosocomial FUO [3,5].

Immune-deficient FUO, also known as neutropenic FUO, is defined as a temperature of 38.3°C (101°F) or greater on several occasions in a patient with a neutrophil count less than 500 cells/μL or expected to reach that level in 1 to 2 days and in whom initial cultures are negative and the diagnosis remains unknown after 3 days of investigation. Frequent causes of neutropenic FUO are perianal infection, aspergillosis, and candidemia [6]. A less common etiology for neutropenic FUO is herpes virus infection.

HIV-associated FUO refers to a temperature of 38.3°C (101°F) or greater on several occasions in an HIV-positive patient. The fever should last for 4 weeks as an outpatient or for 3 days as an inpatient under investigation, including at least 2 days for cultures to incubate. *Mycobacterium avium intracellulare* (MAI), tuberculosis, *Pneumocystis carinii* pneumonia, and cytomegalovirus (CMV) are common causes of HIV-associated FUO. Noninfectious causes, such as lymphoma, Kaposi's sarcoma, and drug fever, are less common [6,7].

The previously mentioned classification is used mostly in the adult population. In children, several studies have defined FUO in children as a fever that lasts 1 to 3 weeks without diagnosis [8–12]. The current definition that is used by most pediatricians is a fever of at least 8 days' duration, in which no diagnosis is apparent after an initial workup in the hospital or as an outpatient. FUO in children has to be differentiated from fever without localizing signs. In the latter, there is development of additional clinical manifestations over a shorter period that leads to less extensive diagnostic testing before confirming the nature of the disease.

Differential diagnosis

The differential diagnosis of FUO is generally divided into four major groups: infections, malignancies, aseptic inflammatory diseases (eg, granulomatous diseases, collagen vascular diseases), and miscellaneous causes [Table 1]. Infections, malignancies, and noninfectious inflammatory diseases account for most classic FUO cases [1,13–15]. After malignancy overtook infection during the 1970s, infection has re-emerged as the most common cause of FUO, accounting for approximately one third of the cases [4,13,16]. Currently, malignancy is the second most frequent category in adults, followed by aseptic inflammatory disease [15,17]. In children, infection is the most common etiology of FUO (30%–50% of cases), followed by connective tissue diseases and then malignancy (7%–13%) [10,11]. In prolonged FUO, malignancy and factitious fever are more likely than other etiologies [18].

Table 1: **Common causes of fever of unknown origin**

Infections	Malignancies	Inflammatory diseases	Miscellaneous
Tuberculosis	Lymphoma	Adult Still's disease	Drug-induced fever
Abdominal	Chronic leukemia	Polymyalgia rheumatica	Central nervous
abscesses	Renal cell carcinoma	Temporal arteritis	dysautonomia
Pelvic abscesses	Metastatic cancers	Rheumatoid arthritis	Deep venous thrombosis
Endocarditis	Colon carcinoma	Inflammatory bowel disease	Periodic fevers
Osteomyelitis	Hepatoma	Systemic lupus erythematosus	Pulmonary embolism
Sinusitis	Pancreatic carcinoma	Vasculitides	Diabetes insipidus
Cytomegalovirus	Sarcomas	Juvenile idiopathic arthritis	Familial dysautonomia
Epstein-Barr virus	Myelodysplastic		Serum sickness
HIV	syndromes		Infantile cortical
Lyme disease	Neuroblastoma		hyperostosis
Prostatitis	Wilms' tumor		Factitious fever

The causes of FUO reported in the literature have differed among various patient groups according to geographic locations, immunologic status, age, and times of the reports, mostly because of dramatic improvements in diagnostic tools. For example, temporal arteritis, tumors, and tuberculosis are more likely in older persons than in younger ones, but self-limited viral syndromes are more common in children [19,20]. In HIV-infected patients, FUO is almost always attributable to an infectious source [7]. The differential diagnosis of FUO is wider in travelers, who may be exposed to unusual infectious agents that they bring with them when they return home [21].

Infections

Tuberculosis and abdominal or pelvic abscesses are the most common infectious diseases associated with FUO in adults [22]. Other frequent causes include sinusitis, subacute bacterial endocarditis, osteomyelitis, and dental abscess [15,22]. Conversely, salmonellosis, rickettsial infections, spirochetal infections, cat-scratch disease, infectious mononucleosis, CMV infection, and viral hepatitis are the most common systemic infections in children with FUO.

Malignancies

In adults and children, lymphoma (especially non-Hodgkin's lymphoma [NHL]) and leukemia are the most common malignancies to present as FUO, but their frequency is decreasing according to two series, which was attributed to improved diagnostic techniques [14,23]. The common solid tumors that cause FUO are renal cell carcinoma and hepatocellular carcinoma or other tumors metastatic to the liver [16].

Noninfectious inflammatory diseases

When collagen vascular diseases and granulomatous diseases were grouped together, this category was found to be more a common cause of FUO than tumors [14,15]. In young adults (<50 years old), systemic-onset juvenile rheumatoid arthritis (JRA; formerly called Still's disease) is the most frequent diagnosis [13–15,22]. In older adults, however, giant cell arteritis is the most common rheumatologic disorder presenting as FUO and represents approximately 15% of the cases [19,24,25]. JRA (now called juvenile idiopathic arthritis [JIA]) is common in children, whereas systemic lupus erythematosus (SLE), Wegener's granulomatosis, and polyarteritis nodosa are more common in adults [10,20,26].

Miscellaneous

In this category, the most common cause of FUO is drug-induced fever, which constitutes a form of hypersensitivity to specific drugs [15]. Deep venous thrombosis (DVT) should be considered in relevant patients [17].

Evaluation of the patient with fever of unknown origin by conventional methods

FUO remains a challenging clinical problem despite advances in investigative tools. The initial approach to the patient with FUO is to take a careful comprehensive history, perform a complete physical examination, and reassess the patient frequently.

The initial assessment of a patient with FUO includes a complete blood cell count with differential, erythrocyte sedimentation rate (ESR), routine chemistry tests (including liver enzymes), urinalysis, basic cultures, and a chest radiograph. The preliminary evaluation helps in the formulation of a differential diagnosis. A subsequent workup, including serology, ultrasonography (US), CT, MRI, and nuclear medicine scanning, should be guided by abnormalities found on the initial assessment so as to avoid haphazard use of invasive and expensive tests.

Radiographic evaluation

After the regular chest radiograph, further radiographic examination of specific areas, such as the nasal sinuses and mastoids, should be performed, especially in children. Echocardiograms are useful in the evaluation for atrial myxoma or endocarditis [27]. US is a low-cost test that can detect fluid collections, abscesses, and DVT and permits the evaluation of the kidneys, pancreas, pelvis, and hepatobiliary tract [28,29]. CT and MRI are useful to rule out such causes of FUO as neoplasms, abscesses, hematomas, lymphadenopathy related to lymphoma or granulomatous diseases, mastoiditis, and vasculitis [30,31]. MRI is preferred if a paraspinal lesion is suspected [32].

General nuclear medicine

Technetium-99m– or indium-111–labeled white blood cells can be helpful in localizing abscesses and osteoarticular infections [33,34]. Gallium-67–citrate scintigraphy (GS) is useful in detecting infectious and inflammatory processes as well as certain tumors, such as lymphoma [35,36]. Other radiopharmaceutic agents that are being studied for potential clinical use in patients with FUO are avidin-labeled biotin, radiolabeled liposomes, labeled cytokines, labeled antibiotics, and labeled monoclonal antibodies [37–40].

18-Fluoro-2-deoxyglucose PET

The latest diagnostic imaging technique in the evaluation of patients with FUO is PET). Although the availability of PET scans is still somewhat limited, it seems to be a useful diagnostic tool in the evaluation of patients with FUO, with a high negative predictive value in ruling out inflammatory and malignant causes of fever.

Mechanism of action

18-Fluoro-2-deoxyglucose (FDG) initially follows the same pathway as glucose. It is transported into the cell by glucose transporters and then phosphorylated by hexokinase. After being phosphorylated, however, FDG remains trapped inside the cell, which enables us to image glucose metabolism in the body [41]. Enhanced glycolysis in malignant cells and activated leukocytes leads to a higher concentration of FDG in the cytoplasm [42]. This is related to high intracellular enzyme levels of hexokinase, increased expression of surface glucose transporter proteins, and a high affinity of these transporters for FDG [41,43–45]. Recent experimental studies have demonstrated the high retention of FDG in inflammatory as well as malignant lesions [46].

Basis for the use of 18-fluoro-2-deoxyglucose PET in fever of unknown origin

FDG, which is currently the most clinically used radiotracer in PET, is not tumor specific. The non-specificity of FDG is of great value in the setting of FUO because it accumulates in inflammation as well as malignancies, which are the most common categories of FUO. FDG-PET has proven to be an accurate imaging modality for the evaluation of a variety of malignancies, such as lymphoma, lung cancer, colorectal cancer, malignant melanoma, head and neck cancer, and breast cancer [47].

FDG can also accumulate in sites of many types of inflammation and infection [48–57]. Therefore, there is an increasing amount of data addressing the value of FDG-PET in the detection of infectious and/or inflammatory processes [58,59]. In the concept of detecting the source of FUO, the low specificity of FDG is, in fact, an advantage attributable to the diversity of causes of the FUO. FDG-PET can be used for diagnosing diabetes-related infections, especially in the evaluation of the diabetic foot [60]; identification of vascular graft infection [61,62]; diagnosis of infection in patients with multiple myeloma [63]; and early detection of bone infection and differentiation from postsurgical inflammation [64–66].

In HIV-associated FUO, the patients are prone to opportunistic infections and malignancies, especially lymphoma. It was shown that a half-body FDG-PET scan had a sensitivity of 92% and a specificity of 94% for localization of focal pathologic findings that needed treatment in patients with HIV [67]. FDG-PET could be helpful in differentiating lymphoma from nonmalignant lesions, such as toxoplasmosis and neurosyphilis, in the central nervous system in HIV-positive patients because of different FDG uptake levels [68].

It is sometimes difficult for FDG-PET to distinguish between aseptic inflammatory disease and infections or malignancies; however, this low specificity is not a disadvantage in classic FUO, because localization of the active lesions in the body would permit a biopsy or evaluation by other imaging modalities. This is the case, for example, with granulomatous diseases, such as sarcoidosis or tuberculosis and lymphoma [69,70]. Conversely, FDG-PET has demonstrated a high sensitivity in detecting autoimmune diseases, such as large-vessel vasculitis [71,72], inflammatory bowel disease [73,74], and inflammatory arthritis. Other examples of infectious or inflammatory process that can be detected with FDG-PET are DVT [75], deep septic thrombophlebitis [76], and infected implantable devices [77]. Various infectious and aseptic inflammatory diseases detected by FDG-PET are presented in Table 2.

18-Fluoro-2-deoxyglucose PET versus other nuclear medicine techniques

Gallium-67–citrate, labeled leukocytes with technetium-99m or indium-111, and FDG represent the most intensely investigated radiopharmaceutic agents in the field of FUO. Because of its availability, low cost, and ability to detect inflammation and malignancy, GS is still the most commonly used radiotracer for the evaluation of FUO [36].

Table 2: Common causes of infectious and NIID detected by 18-fluoro-2-deoxyglucose PET

Infections	NIID
Tuberculosis	Giant cell arteritis
Subphrenic abscess	Takayasu arteritis
Pneumonia	Juvenile idiopathic
Osteomyelitis	arthritis
Vascular graft	Rheumatoid arthritis
infection	Wegener's
Sinusitis	granulomatosis
Mastoiditis	Thyroiditis
Septic	Myositis
thrombophlebitis	Gastritis
Abdominal abscess	Noninfectious
Diverticulitis	encephalitis
Infected joint	Pleuritis
prosthesis	Inflammatory bowel
Cellulitis	disease
	Foreign body–induced
	granuloma

Abbreviation: NIID, non-infectious inflammatory disease.

FDG-PET has many advantages over conventional nuclear medicine techniques, however, because FDG has better tracer kinetics, a favorable 110-minute half-life, and a lower dose to the patient. This allows whole-body FDG-PET scanning to be completed in approximately 2 hours from the injection. This results in earlier reporting than with other radiotracers [78], thus decreasing the frustration of the clinicians who sometimes have to wait 2 to 3 or even 4 days for the results of conventional nuclear medicine techniques. FDG-PET has a better spatial resolution (5–8-mm resolution for PET versus 10–15-mm resolution for single photon emission computed tomography [SPECT]) and a better lesion-to-background ratio [78]. There is also the opportunity with FDG-PET for semi-quantification by the use of standardized uptake values (SUVs), thus decreasing the variability among readers. In addition, handling of FDG is safe, in contrast to labeled leukocytes, because there is no handling of blood products with FDG.

FDG-PET was found to be superior to indium-111–labeled leukocytes, and antigranulocyte antibody scintigraphy in the detection of chronic osteomyelitis, especially in the central skeleton [79,80]. It is more sensitive in chronic low-grade infections [81]. In a recent study on the value of FDG-PET in metastatic infectious disease, FDG-PET detected a clinically relevant new infectious focus in 45% of cases and confirmed lesions already diagnosed in 30% of cases, with a positive predictive value of 91% and a negative predictive value of 100% [82].

In patients with vasculitis, FDG is superior to other radiotracers that occasionally yield a positive result in patients with vasculitis [83]. FDG-PET can detect and evaluate the degree of activity in a variety of inflammatory vessel diseases, especially large-vessel vasculitis [71,84,85]. This is mostly important in the case of temporal arteritis and polymyalgia rheumatica, the most common causes of FUO in the elderly [78,86,87]. Recent studies have also shown that FDG-PET can clearly detect sarcoidosis in the heart, lungs, and brain, whereas concurrent gallium scans are negative [88,89].

GS has been the best available functional imaging modality for evaluating patients with NHL and Hodgkin's disease (HD) until recently. Comparative reports in the past several years have shown that FDG-PET is superior to GS for the detection of nodal and extranodal lymphoma [90–92].

In summary, in cases of classic FUO, it is preferable to use FDG rather than gallium-67 as a nonspecific radiotracer that may spot infection, tumor, or inflammation [93]. In general, FDG-PET is superior to GS because it has a better overall sensitivity without the loss of specificity. In nosocomial FUO, a radiotracer that is more specific for infection, such as labeled leukocytes, might be used [35]. In cases of neutropenic and HIV-associated FUO, however, a nonspecific radiotracer is recommended, preferably FDG over gallium.

Preliminary results indicated that FDG-labeled white blood cells gave better results than FDG when studying sterile and septic inflammation models as part of an experimental study [94]. Another experimental study suggested the feasibility of gallium-68 PET imaging of bone infections [95]. FDG-labeled white cells and gallium-68 might be applied in the detection of the source of FUO. More investigations are necessary to confirm the validity of these new methods, however.

18-Fluoro-2-deoxyglucose PET versus anatomic imaging

Because most cases of FUO reflect unusual manifestations of common diseases, pattern recognition is sometimes of limited value in the diagnostic process. FDG-PET can assess the whole body in one study, which allows the localization of lesions based on functional changes of tissues. CT, MRI, and US are less suitable as a screening method when clues for specific sites of infection or malignancy are absent.

Whole-body scintigraphy in FUO has a role in localizing suspicious areas, which can then be investigated further by US, classic radiographic studies, CT, MRI, endoscopy, or, eventually, biopsy [35].

Conventional anatomic imaging modalities provide excellent anatomic details but rely on size as a criterion to distinguish between malignant and benign diseases. Anatomic imaging has limited capacity in detecting early changes at the molecular level [Fig. 1]. In surgical or orthopedic patients, FDG-PET has an advantage over anatomic imaging. For example, in patients who have fractures, or after surgical intervention, FDG-PET can differentiate between normal bone healing and postsurgical inflammation from osteomyelitis [65,66]. In patients with prostheses, FDG-PET can detect a superimposed infection, especially in hip prostheses [96] and, to a lesser extent, in knee prostheses [97], in contrast to CT and MRI, which are hindered by metal implants [98,99]. Deep septic thrombophlebitis can be identified with FDG-PET in areas not optimally visualized by duplex scan or venography [76]. In a study on patients with multiple myeloma, FDG-PET findings identified infections not detectable by other methods, determined the extent of infection, and led to modifications of workup and therapy [63].

The widespread availability and routine use of anatomic imaging, especially CT, have led to earlier

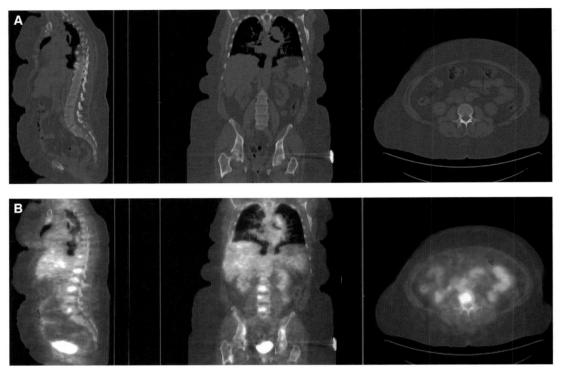

Fig. 1. CT (*A*) and PET-CT (*B*) three-view images of a 49-year-old patient who was evaluated for a suspicious lung nodule and fever. There are multiple foci of abnormal FDG uptake in the spine and pelvis consistent with hypermetabolism in the bone marrow, with no corresponding anatomic abnormalities on CT.

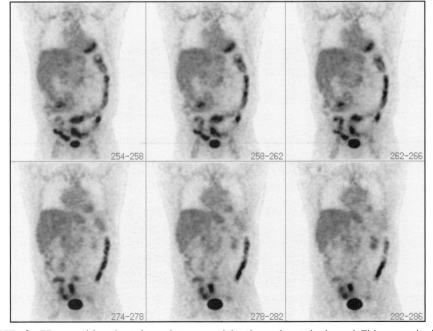

Fig. 2. FDG-PET of a 75-year-old patient shows intense activity throughout the bowel. This example demonstrates how normal bowel activity can sometimes hinder the detection of subtle abnormalities in the intestines.

diagnosis of many tumors, and they are not as common a cause of FUO as they once were. Nevertheless, in cases in which there is no diagnosis obtained from CT or MRI, an FDG-PET scan may identify a tumor.

FDG-PET also has a good safety profile. The radiation dose received by the patient [100], radiocontrast-induced nephropathy [101], and allergic reactions [102] to patients imaged with CT should be taken into consideration, especially in the pediatric population when ordering serial CT scans.

Finally, the combination of anatomic imaging and FDG-PET through coregistration of the images or a combined PET-CT scan allows better localization of functional abnormalities and can be used to guide biopsies to the metabolically active area [103]. This approach has the potential to reduce the sampling error, morbidity, cost, and the need for unnecessary invasive procedures.

Limitations of 18-fluoro-2-deoxyglucose PET

Certain areas of the body can sometimes be difficult to evaluate because of the normally high FDG

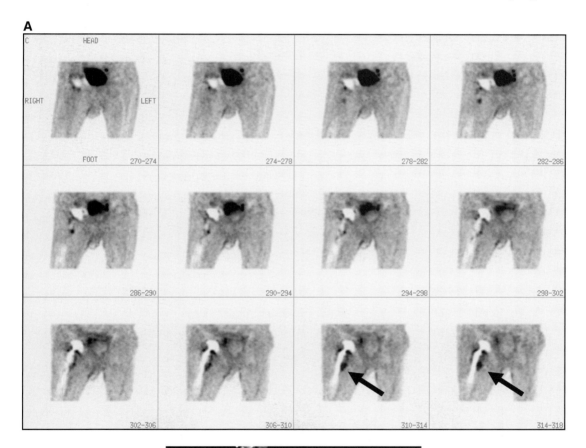

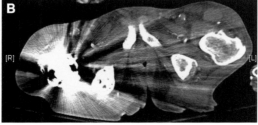

Fig. 3. An 86-year-old patient who was admitted to the hospital for FUO and mental status change. (*A*) After an extensive negative workup, the patient underwent a PET scan that revealed abnormal activity around the shaft of the right hip prosthesis consistent with a periprosthetic infection (*arrows*). (*B*) Patient had a CT scan of the abdomen and pelvis as part of the workup, but the metal artifact prevented the evaluation of the right hip prosthesis.

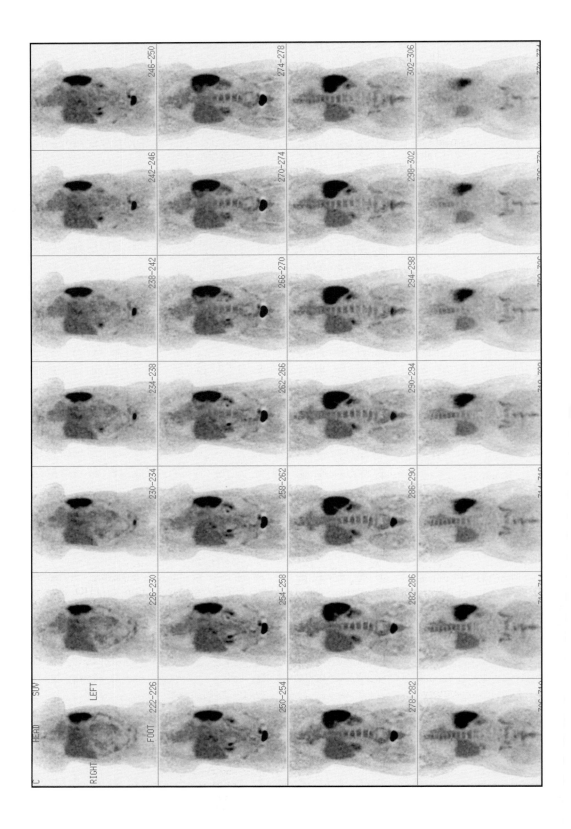

activity in the kidneys, urinary tract, bladder, brain, and myocardium. The accuracy of FDG-PET in the evaluation of the abdomen can also be decreased by the variable intensity in the bowel [Fig. 2]. This issue seems to be less concerning in pediatric patients, in whom there is usually low FDG activity in the bowel [104]. Familiarity with the normal distribution of FDG throughout the body and the variations that might occur with age is necessary to interpret FDG-PET images accurately. Potential pitfalls in sensitivity and false-negative findings on FDG-PET can occur in lesions less than 1 cm in diameter [105,106] and in tumors with low metabolic activity, such as carcinoid [107], broncho-alveolar cell carcinoma [108,109], hepatocellular carcinoma [110,111], certain pancreatic tumors [112], and low-grade cartilaginous tumors [113]. Although FDG-PET can readily visualize large vessel vasculitis, it remains less effective in the detection of small vessel disease.

Intense physical activity, abnormal blood sugar levels, or the administration of insulin just before the injection of FDG can hinder the quality of the images. We have reported that the detection of inflammatory and infectious lesions is not necessarily affected by serum glucose levels, however [114]. Other disadvantages of FDG-PET are the relatively high cost and the currently limited availability.

18-Fluoro-2-deoxyglucose PET and fever of unknown origin in the literature

Overall, investigators have reported that FDG-PET scans were helpful in the diagnosis of FUO in 37% to 69% of patients [78,115–119]. This great variation is attributed to varying definitions of FUO, a wide array of heterogeneous disorders, different FDG-PET techniques (dedicated PET versus dual-head coincidence cameras), and lack of a structured diagnostic protocol. Because of the low specificity of FDG-PET in a patient with FUO and the difficulty in obtaining proof for the assessment of scintigraphic methods, Peters [35] suggested changing the term *true-positive scintigraphy* to *useful-positive scintigraphy*. Knockaert and colleagues [93] classified positive results in their studies on the diagnostic contribution of scintigraphic methods in FUO as diagnostically helpful or diagnostically noncontributory.

Blockmans and coworkers [78] studied 58 consecutive cases of FUO comparing FDG-PET with GS and reported that FDG-PET was helpful in the diagnosis more often than GS (35% versus 25%, respectively). When comparing a dual-head coincidence FDG-PET scan with GS, Meller and colleagues [115] found that FDG-PET contributed to a diagnosis in 55% of the 20 prospective studies. FDG-PET using a dual-head coincidence PET camera was superior to GS [115].

Lorenzen and coworkers [116] found a high negative predictive value of FDG-PET in the setting of FUO, because no morphologic origin of the fever could be determined in the patients with a negative FDG-PET scan.

Bleeker-Rovers and colleagues [117] verified that FDG-PET was more helpful in the diagnosis of patients with a suspected focal infection or localized inflammation than in FUO.

Buysschaert and coworkers [118] studied the data from 110 prospectively recruited patients who fulfilled the revised criteria of classic FUO. In their study, 19 FDG-PET scans (36% of the abnormal scans or 26% of the total number of scans) were helpful in the diagnosis. In the 39 patients with a final diagnosis, 49% of the scans were helpful [118].

At our institution, we retrospectively reviewed 31 FDG-PET scans of 31 patients (aged 14–86 years) who were evaluated for FUO during the period between 1999 and 2004. Among the 31 patients, only 18 had a final diagnosis. FDG-PET contributed to the diagnosis in 13 (72%) of the 18 patients. The etiologies for FUO were pneumonia, periprosthetic infection [Fig. 3], NHL, HD, Crohn's disease, surgical wound infection, infected liver cysts, splenic involvement attributable to leukemia [Fig. 4], cholangitis [Fig. 5], and metastatic renal carcinoma. FDG-PET was not contributory in 3 (17%) of the 17 patients, and these patients were finally diagnosed with colitis, peritonitis, and rejected renal transplant. In 2 patients, FDG-PET was falsely positive in the abdomen [Fig. 6].

Not every publication regarding the utility of FDG-PET in the evaluation of FUO is positive. Based on the result of a study of 19 patients, Kjaer and coworkers [119] reported that indium-111–granulocyte scintigraphy has a superior diagnostic performance compared with FDG-PET for detection of an infectious and/or inflammatory or neoplastic cause of FUO. Among the 19 patients studied, however, only 1 was diagnosed with malignancy (HD). In addition, in this investigation, most false interpretations of FDG-PET images were confirmed by "clinical course" only. Therefore, further

Fig. 4. Intense FDG uptake by a moderately enlarged spleen in an immunosuppressed patient with pancytopenia and FUO. A bone marrow biopsy did not demonstrate overt findings to explain the patient's pancytopenia. Flow cytometry on the peripheral blood detected abnormal T lymphocytes. FDG-PET was helpful in guiding the investigation, and the final diagnosis was T-cell lymphoma with splenic involvement.

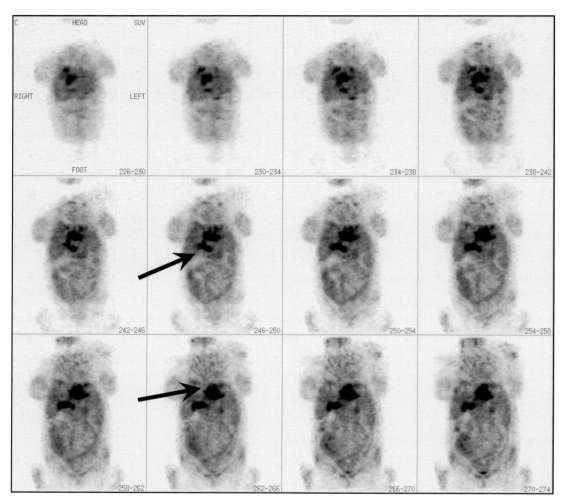

Fig. 5. Coronal views of FDG-PET in a patient with FUO demonstrate abnormal activity in the liver (*arrows*). The study helped the clinician to focus the investigation on the liver, and the patient was eventually diagnosed with cholangitis secondary to Caroli's disease.

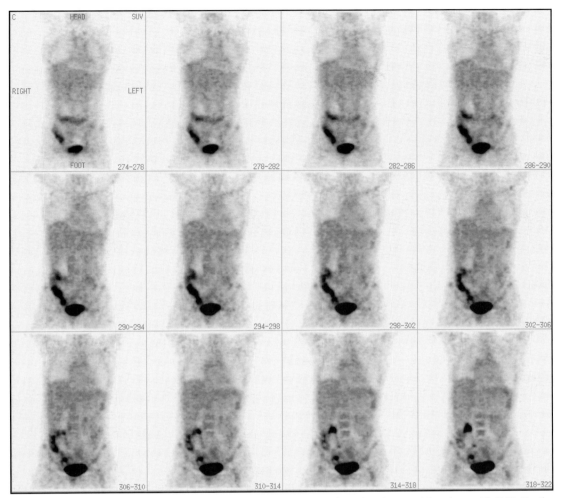

Fig. 6. Intense FDG uptake is seen in the ascending and transverse colon of a 48-year-old patient with FUO. Further investigation, including a tissue biopsy of the colon, was negative for any intestinal pathologic findings. The patient had a final diagnosis of mixed gram-negative intravenous line infection.

investigation involving larger patient populations is necessary to verify this result.

Summary

FDG-PET is a valuable new imaging technique that has major advantages over conventional nuclear medicine and anatomic imaging techniques for the assessment of patients with FUO. FDG-PET can detect a great number of malignancies as well as infectious and aseptic inflammatory diseases, which account for most FUO etiologies. The high diagnostic yield of FDG-PET adds valuable clinical information that can be used to focus the investigation of FUO. By evaluating the whole body and obtaining adequate early diagnosis, it limits the number of unnecessary procedures and the time to diagnosis and thus facilitates prompt and adequate therapy.

References

[1] Petersdorf RG, Beeson PB. Fever of unexplained origin: report on 100 cases. Medicine (Baltimore) 1961;40:1–30.

[2] Durack DT, Street AC. Fever of unknown origin—reexamined and redefined. Curr Clin Top Infect Dis 1991;11:35–51.

[3] Konecny P, Davidson RN. Pyrexia of unknown origin in the 1990s: time to redefine. Br J Hosp Med 1996;56:21–4.

[4] Petersdorf RG. Fever of unknown origin. An old friend revisited. Arch Intern Med 1992;152: 21–2.

[5] Kountakis SE, Burke L, Rafie JJ, et al. Sinusitis

in the intensive care unit patient. Otolaryngol Head Neck Surg 1997;117:362–6.

[6] Hughes WT, Armstrong D, Bodey GP, et al. 1997 guidelines for the use of antimicrobial agents in neutropenic patients with unexplained fever. Infectious Diseases Society of America. Clin Infect Dis 1997;25:551–73.

[7] Armstrong WS, Katz JT, Kazanjian PH. Human immunodeficiency virus-associated fever of unknown origin: a study of 70 patients in the United States and review. Clin Infect Dis 1999; 28:341–5.

[8] McClung HJ. Prolonged fever of unknown origin in children. Am J Dis Child 1972;124: 544–50.

[9] Dechovitz AB, Moffet HL. Classification of acute febrile illnesses in childhood. Clin Pediatr (Phila) 1968;7:649–53.

[10] Pizzo PA, Lovejoy Jr FH, Smith DH. Prolonged fever in children: review of 100 cases. Pediatrics 1975;55:468–73.

[11] Lohr JA, Hendley JO. Prolonged fever of unknown origin: a record of experiences with 54 childhood patients. Clin Pediatr (Phila) 1977; 16:768–73.

[12] Brewis EG. Child care in general practice. Undiagnosed fever. BMJ 1965;5427:107–9.

[13] Larson EB, Featherstone HJ, Petersdorf RG. Fever of undetermined origin: diagnosis and follow-up of 105 cases, 1970–1980. Medicine (Baltimore) 1982;61:269–92.

[14] Knockaert DC, Vanneste LJ, Vanneste SB, et al. Fever of unknown origin in the 1980s. An update of the diagnostic spectrum. Arch Intern Med 1992;152:51–5.

[15] de Kleijn EM, Vandenbroucke JP, van der Meer JW. Fever of unknown origin (FUO). I. A prospective multicenter study of 167 patients with FUO, using fixed epidemiologic entry criteria. The Netherlands FUO Study Group. Medicine (Baltimore) 1997;76:392–400.

[16] Knockaert DC, Vanneste LJ, Bobbaers HJ. Recurrent or episodic fever of unknown origin. Review of 45 cases and survey of the literature. Medicine (Baltimore) 1993;72:184–96.

[17] Mourad O, Palda V, Detsky AS. A comprehensive evidence-based approach to fever of unknown origin. Arch Intern Med 2003;163: 545–51.

[18] Aduan RP, Fauci AS, Dale DC, et al. Factitious fever and self-induced infection: a report of 32 cases and review of the literature. Ann Intern Med 1979;90:230–42.

[19] Tal S, Guller V, Gurevich A, et al. Fever of unknown origin in the elderly. J Intern Med 2002; 252:295–304.

[20] Knockaert DC, Vanneste LJ, Bobbaers HJ. Fever of unknown origin in elderly patients. J Am Geriatr Soc 1993;41:1187–92.

[21] Strickland GT. Fever in the returned traveler. Med Clin North Am 1992;76:1375–92.

[22] Kazanjian PH. Fever of unknown origin: review

of 86 patients treated in community hospitals. Clin Infect Dis 1992;15:968–73.

[23] Iikuni Y, Okada J, Kondo H, et al. Current fever of unknown origin 1982–1992. Intern Med 1994;33:67–73.

[24] Hirschmann JV. Fever of unknown origin in adults. Clin Infect Dis 1997;24:291–300 [quiz: 301–2].

[25] Arnow PM, Flaherty JP. Fever of unknown origin. Lancet 1997;350:575–80.

[26] Cunha BA. Fever of unknown origin. Infect Dis Clin North Am 1996;10:111–27.

[27] Hoen B, Beguinot I, Rabaud C, et al. The Duke criteria for diagnosing infective endocarditis are specific: analysis of 100 patients with acute fever or fever of unknown origin. Clin Infect Dis 1996;23:298–302.

[28] Picardi M, Morante R, Rotoli B. Ultrasound exploration in the work-up of unexplained fever in the immunocompromised host: preliminary observations. Haematologica 1997;82:455–7.

[29] Abu Rahma AF, Saiedy S, Robinson PA, et al. Role of venous duplex imaging of the lower extremities in patients with fever of unknown origin. Surgery 1997;121:366–71.

[30] Cheng MF, Chiou CC, Hsieh KS. Mastoiditis: a disease often overlooked by pediatricians. J Microbiol Immunol Infect 2000;33:237–40.

[31] Wagner AD, Andresen J, Raum E, et al. Standardised work-up programme for fever of unknown origin and contribution of magnetic resonance imaging for the diagnosis of hidden systemic vasculitis. Ann Rheum Dis 2005;64: 105–10.

[32] Bluman EM, Palumbo MA, Lucas PR. Spinal epidural abscess in adults. J Am Acad Orthop Surg 2004;12:155–63.

[33] Kjaer A, Lebech AM. Diagnostic value of (111) In-granulocyte scintigraphy in patients with fever of unknown origin. J Nucl Med 2002;43: 140–4.

[34] Peters AM. The utility of [99mTc]HMPAO-leukocytes for imaging infection. Semin Nucl Med 1994;24:110–27.

[35] Peters AM. Nuclear medicine imaging in fever of unknown origin. Q J Nucl Med 1999;43: 61–73.

[36] Knockaert DC, Mortelmans LA, De Roo MC, et al. Clinical value of gallium-67 scintigraphy in evaluation of fever of unknown origin. Clin Infect Dis 1994;18:601–5.

[37] Meller J, Ivancevic V, Conrad M, et al. Clinical value of immunoscintigraphy in patients with fever of unknown origin. J Nucl Med 1998;39: 1248–53.

[38] Maugeri D, Santangelo A, Abbate S, et al. A new method for diagnosing fever of unknown origin (FUO) due to infection of muscular-skeletal system in elderly people: leukoscan Tc-99m labelled scintigraphy. Eur Rev Med Pharmacol Sci 2001;5:123–6.

[39] Gallowitsch HJ, Heinisch M, Mikosch P, et al.

[Tc-99m ciprofloxacin in clinically selected patients for peripheral osteomyelitis, spondylodiscitis and fever of unknown origin—preliminary results]. Nuklearmedizin 2002;41: 30–6 [in German].

[40] Dams ET, Oyen WJ, Boerman OC, et al. 99mTc-PEG liposomes for the scintigraphic detection of infection and inflammation: clinical evaluation. J Nucl Med 2000;41:622–30.

[41] Ak I, Stokkel MP, Pauwels EK. Positron emission tomography with 2-[18F]fluoro-2-deoxy-D-glucose in oncology. Part II. The clinical value in detecting and staging primary tumours. J Cancer Res Clin Oncol 2000;126:560–74.

[42] Kubota R, Yamada S, Kubota K, et al. Intratumoral distribution of fluorine-18-fluorodeoxyglucose in vivo: high accumulation in macrophages and granulation tissues studied by microautoradiography. J Nucl Med 1992;33:1972–80.

[43] Avril N, Menzel M, Dose J, et al. Glucose metabolism of breast cancer assessed by 18F-FDG PET: histologic and immunohistochemical tissue analysis. J Nucl Med 2001;42:9–16.

[44] Chakrabarti R, Jung CY, Lee TP, et al. Changes in glucose transport and transporter isoforms during the activation of human peripheral blood lymphocytes by phytohemagglutinin. J Immunol 1994;152:2660–8.

[45] Ahmed N, Kansara M, Berridge MV. Acute regulation of glucose transport in a monocyte-macrophage cell line: Glut-3 affinity for glucose is enhanced during the respiratory burst. Biochem J 1997;327(Pt 2):369–75.

[46] Kok PJ, van Eerd JE, Boerman OC, et al. Biodistribution and imaging of FDG in rats with LS174T carcinoma xenografts and focal Escherichia coli infection. Cancer Biother Radiopharm 2005;20:310–5.

[47] Kostakoglu L, Agress Jr H, Goldsmith SJ. Clinical role of FDG PET in evaluation of cancer patients. Radiographics 2003;23:315–40 [quiz: 533].

[48] Thomas A, Singh A, Greenspan B. Localization of F-18FDG in Nocardia lung infection. Clin Nucl Med 2004;29:834–5.

[49] Zhuang H, Chacko TK, Hickeson M, et al. Persistent non-specific FDG uptake on PET imaging following hip arthroplasty. Eur J Nucl Med Mol Imag 2002;29:1328–33.

[50] Zhuang H, Cunnane ME, Ghesani NV, et al. Chest tube insertion as a potential source of false-positive FDG-positron emission tomographic results. Clin Nucl Med 2002;27:285–6.

[51] Zhuang H, Duarte PS, Rebenstock A, et al. Pulmonary Clostridium perfringens infection detected by FDG positron emission tomography. Clin Nucl Med 2003;28:517–8.

[52] Nguyen QH, Szeto E, Mansberg R, et al. Paravertebral infection (phlegmon) demonstrated by FDG dual-head coincidence imaging in a patient with multiple malignancies. Clin Nucl Med 2005;30:241–3.

[53] Stadler P, Bilohlavek O, Spacek M, et al. Diagnosis of vascular prosthesis infection with FDG-PET/CT. J Vasc Surg 2004;40:1246–7.

[54] Shin L, Katz DS, Yung E. Hypermetabolism on F-18 FDG PET of multiple pulmonary nodules resulting from bronchiolitis obliterans organizing pneumonia. Clin Nucl Med 2004; 29:654–6.

[55] Hsu CH, Lee CM, Wang FC, et al. F-18 fluorodeoxyglucose positron emission tomography in pulmonary cryptococcoma. Clin Nucl Med 2003;28:791–3.

[56] Schuster DP, Kozlowski J, Hogue L, et al. Imaging lung inflammation in a murine model of Pseudomonas infection: a positron emission tomography study. Exp Lung Res 2003;29:45–57.

[57] Yu JQ, Kumar R, Xiu Y, et al. Diffuse FDG uptake in the lungs in aspiration pneumonia on positron emission tomographic imaging. Clin Nucl Med 2004;29:567–8.

[58] Zhuang H, Alavi A. 18-Fluorodeoxyglucose positron emission tomographic imaging in the detection and monitoring of infection and inflammation. Semin Nucl Med 2002;32:47–59.

[59] El-Haddad G, Zhuang H, Gupta N, et al. Evolving role of positron emission tomography in the management of patients with inflammatory and other benign disorders. Semin Nucl Med 2004;34:313–29.

[60] Keidar Z, Militianu D, Melamed E, et al. The diabetic foot: initial experience with 18F-FDG PET/CT. J Nucl Med 2005;46:444–9.

[61] Fukuchi K, Ishida Y, Higashi M, et al. Detection of aortic graft infection by fluorodeoxyglucose positron emission tomography: comparison with computed tomographic findings. J Vasc Surg 2005;42:919–25.

[62] Krupnick A, Lombardi J, Engels F, et al. 18-Fluorodeoxyglucose positron emission tomography as a novel imaging tool for the diagnosis of aortoenteric fistula and aortic graft infection—a case report. Vasc Endovascular Surg 2003;37:363–8.

[63] Mahfouz T, Miceli MH, Saghafifar F, et al. 18F-fluorodeoxyglucose positron emission tomography contributes to the diagnosis and management of infections in patients with multiple myeloma: a study of 165 infectious episodes. J Clin Oncol 2005;23:7857–63.

[64] Zhuang H, Duarte PS, Pourdehand M, et al. Exclusion of chronic osteomyelitis with F-18 fluorodeoxyglucose positron emission tomographic imaging. Clin Nucl Med 2000;25: 281–4.

[65] Jones-Jackson L, Walker R, Purnell G, et al. Early detection of bone infection and differentiation from post-surgical inflammation using 2-deoxy-2-[18F]-fluoro-D-glucose positron emission tomography (FDG-PET) in an animal model. J Orthop Res 2005;23:1484–9.

[66] Zhuang H, Sam JW, Chacko TK, et al. Rapid normalization of osseous FDG uptake following

traumatic or surgical fractures. Eur J Nucl Med Mol Imaging 2003;30:1096–103.

[67] O'Doherty MJ, Barrington SF, Campbell M, et al. PET scanning and the human immunodeficiency virus-positive patient. J Nucl Med 1997;38:1575–83.

[68] Heald AE, Hoffman JM, Bartlett JA, et al. Differentiation of central nervous system lesions in AIDS patients using positron emission tomography (PET). Int J STD AIDS 1996;7: 337–46.

[69] Barrington SF, O'Doherty MJ. Limitations of PET for imaging lymphoma. Eur J Nucl Med Mol Imaging 2003;30(Suppl 1):S117–27.

[70] Konishi J, Yamazaki K, Tsukamoto E, et al. Mediastinal lymph node staging by FDG-PET in patients with non-small cell lung cancer: analysis of false-positive FDG-PET findings. Respiration (Herrlisheim) 2003;70:500–6.

[71] Walter MA, Melzer RA, Schindler C, et al. The value of [(18)F]FDG-PET in the diagnosis of large-vessel vasculitis and the assessment of activity and extent of disease. Eur J Nucl Med Mol Imaging 2005;32(6):674–81.

[72] Moosig F, Czech N, Mehl C, et al. Correlation between 18-fluorodeoxyglucose accumulation in large vessels and serological markers of inflammation in polymyalgia rheumatica: a quantitative PET study. Ann Rheum Dis 2004; 63:870–3.

[73] Neurath MF, Vehling D, Schunk K, et al. Noninvasive assessment of Crohn's disease activity: a comparison of 18F-fluorodeoxyglucose positron emission tomography, hydromagnetic resonance imaging, and granulocyte scintigraphy with labeled antibodies. Am J Gastroenterol 2002;97:1978–85.

[74] Pio BS, Byrne FR, Aranda R, et al. Noninvasive quantification of bowel inflammation through positron emission tomography imaging of 2-deoxy-2-[18F]fluoro-D-glucose-labeled white blood cells. Mol Imaging Biol 2003;5:271–7.

[75] Chang KJ, Zhuang H, Alavi A. Detection of chronic recurrent lower extremity deep venous thrombosis on fluorine-18 fluorodeoxyglucose positron emission tomography. Clin Nucl Med 2000;25:838–9.

[76] Miceli M, Atoui R, Walker R, et al. Diagnosis of deep septic thrombophlebitis in cancer patients by fluorine-18 fluorodeoxyglucose positron emission tomography scanning: a preliminary report. J Clin Oncol 2004;22:1949–56.

[77] Miceli MH, Jones Jackson LB, Walker RC, et al. Diagnosis of infection of implantable central venous catheters by [18F]fluorodeoxyglucose positron emission tomography. Nucl Med Commun 2004;25:813–8.

[78] Blockmans D, Knockaert D, Maes A, et al. Clinical value of [(18)F]fluoro-deoxyglucose positron emission tomography for patients with fever of unknown origin. Clin Infect Dis 2001; 32:191–6.

[79] Guhlmann A, Brecht-Krauss D, Suger G, et al. Fluorine-18-FDG PET and technetium-99m anti-granulocyte antibody scintigraphy in chronic osteomyelitis. J Nucl Med 1998;39:2145–52.

[80] Meller J, Koster G, Liersch T, et al. Chronic bacterial osteomyelitis: prospective comparison of (18)F-FDG imaging with a dual-head coincidence camera and (111)In-labelled autologous leucocyte scintigraphy. Eur J Nucl Med Mol Imaging 2002;29:53–60.

[81] Guhlmann A, Brecht-Krauss D, Suger G, et al. Chronic osteomyelitis: detection with FDG PET and correlation with histopathologic findings. Radiology 1998;206:749–54.

[82] Bleeker-Rovers CP, Vos FJ, Wanten GJ, et al. 18F-FDG PET in detecting metastatic infectious disease. J Nucl Med 2005;46:2014–9.

[83] Jonker ND, Peters AM, Gaskin G, et al. A retrospective study of radiolabeled granulocyte kinetics in patients with systemic vasculitis. J Nucl Med 1992;33:491–7.

[84] Salvarani C, Pipitone N, Versari A, et al. Positron emission tomography (PET): evaluation of chronic periaortitis. Arthritis Rheum 2005;53: 298–303.

[85] Kobayashi Y, Ishii K, Oda K, et al. Aortic wall inflammation due to Takayasu arteritis imaged with 18F-FDG PET coregistered with enhanced CT. J Nucl Med 2005;46:917–22.

[86] Blockmans D, Stroobants S, Maes A, et al. Positron emission tomography in giant cell arteritis and polymyalgia rheumatica: evidence for inflammation of the aortic arch. Am J Med 2000; 108:246–9.

[87] Turlakow A, Yeung HW, Pui J, et al. Fludeoxyglucose positron emission tomography in the diagnosis of giant cell arteritis. Arch Intern Med 2001;161:1003–7.

[88] Ishimaru S, Tsujino I, Takei T, et al. Focal uptake on 18F-fluoro-2-deoxyglucose positron emission tomography images indicates cardiac involvement of sarcoidosis. Eur Heart J 2005;26: 1538–43.

[89] Xiu Y, Yu JQ, Cheng E, et al. Sarcoidosis demonstrated by FDG PET imaging with negative findings on gallium scintigraphy. Clin Nucl Med 2005;30:193–5.

[90] Kostakoglu L, Leonard JP, Kuji I, et al. Comparison of fluorine-18 fluorodeoxyglucose positron emission tomography and Ga-67 scintigraphy in evaluation of lymphoma. Cancer 2002;94: 879–88.

[91] Lin P, Chu J, Kneebone A, et al. Direct comparison of 18F-fluorodeoxyglucose coincidence gamma camera tomography with gallium scanning for the staging of lymphoma. Intern Med J 2005;35:91–6.

[92] Yamamoto F, Tsukamoto E, Nakada K, et al. 18F-FDG PET is superior to 67Ga SPECT in the staging of non-Hodgkin's lymphoma. Ann Nucl Med 2004;18:519–26.

[93] Knockaert DC, Vanderschueren S, Blockmans D.

Fever of unknown origin in adults: 40 years on. J Intern Med 2003;253:263–75.

[94] Pellegrino D, Bonab AA, Dragotakes SC, et al. Inflammation and infection: imaging properties of 18F-FDG-labeled white blood cells versus 18F-FDG. J Nucl Med 2005;46:1522–30.

[95] Makinen TJ, Lankinen P, Poyhonen T, et al. Comparison of (18)F-FDG and (68)Ga PET imaging in the assessment of experimental osteomyelitis due to Staphylococcus aureus. Eur J Nucl Med Mol Imaging 2005;32:1259–68.

[96] Chacko TK, Zhuang H, Stevenson K, et al. The importance of the location of fluorodeoxyglucose uptake in periprosthetic infection in painful hip prostheses. Nucl Med Commun 2002; 23:851–5.

[97] Zhuang H, Duarte PS, Pourdehnad M, et al. The promising role of 18F-FDG PET in detecting infected lower limb prosthesis implants. J Nucl Med 2001;42:44–8.

[98] Erdman WA, Tamburro F, Jayson HT, et al. Osteomyelitis: characteristics and pitfalls of diagnosis with MR imaging. Radiology 1991; 180:533–9.

[99] Crim JR, Seeger LL. Imaging evaluation of osteomyelitis. Crit Rev Diagn Imaging 1994;35: 201–56.

[100] Buls N, de Mey J, Covens P, et al. Health screening with CT: prospective assessment of radiation dose and associated detriment. JBR-BTR 2005;88:12–6.

[101] Asif A, Epstein M. Prevention of radiocontrast-induced nephropathy. Am J Kidney Dis 2004; 44:12–24.

[102] Cochran ST. Anaphylactoid reactions to radio-contrast media. Curr Allergy Asthma Rep 2005; 5:28–31.

[103] Yap JT, Carney JP, Hall NC, et al. Image-guided cancer therapy using PET/CT. Cancer J 2004;10: 221–33.

[104] El-Haddad G, Alavi A, Mavi A, et al. Normal variants in [18F]-fluorodeoxyglucose PET imaging. Radiol Clin North Am 2004;42:1063–81.

[105] Duhaylongsod FG, Lowe VJ, Patz Jr EF, et al. Detection of primary and recurrent lung cancer by means of F-18 fluorodeoxyglucose positron emission tomography (FDG PET). J Thorac Cardiovasc Surg 1995;110:130–9 [discussion: 139–40].

[106] Gupta NC, Frank AR, Dewan NA, et al. Solitary pulmonary nodules: detection of malignancy with PET with 2-[F-18]-fluoro-2-deoxy-D-glucose. Radiology 1992;184:441–4.

[107] Erasmus JJ, McAdams HP, Patz Jr EF, et al. Evaluation of primary pulmonary carcinoid tumors using FDG PET. AJR Am J Roentgenol 1998;170:1369–73.

[108] Higashi K, Ueda Y, Seki H, et al. Fluorine-18-FDG PET imaging is negative in bronchiolo-alveolar lung carcinoma. J Nucl Med 1998;39: 1016–20.

[109] Scott WJ, Schwabe JL, Gupta NC, et al. Positron emission tomography of lung tumors and mediastinal lymph nodes using [18F]fluoro-deoxyglucose. The members of the PET-Lung Tumor Study Group. Ann Thorac Surg 1994;58: 698–703.

[110] Torizuka T, Tamaki N, Inokuma T, et al. In vivo assessment of glucose metabolism in hepato-cellular carcinoma with FDG-PET. J Nucl Med 1995;36:1811–7.

[111] Lee JD, Yang WI, Park YN, et al. Different glucose uptake and glycolytic mechanisms between hepatocellular carcinoma and intra-hepatic mass-forming cholangiocarcinoma with increased (18)F-FDG uptake. J Nucl Med 2005; 46:1753–9.

[112] Delbeke D, Pinson CW. Pancreatic tumors: role of imaging in the diagnosis, staging, and treatment. J Hepatobiliary Pancreat Surg 2004; 11:4–10.

[113] Lee FY, Yu J, Chang SS, et al. Diagnostic value and limitations of fluorine-18 fluorodeoxyglu-cose positron emission tomography for cartilagi-nous tumors of bone. J Bone Joint Surg Am 2004;86:2677–85.

[114] Zhuang HM, Cortes-Blanco A, Pourdehnad M, et al. Do high glucose levels have differential effect on FDG uptake in inflammatory and malignant disorders? Nucl Med Commun 2001; 22:1123–8.

[115] Meller J, Altenvoerde G, Munzel U, et al. Fever of unknown origin: prospective comparison of [18F]FDG imaging with a double-head coin-cidence camera and gallium-67 citrate SPET. Eur J Nucl Med 2000;27:1617–25.

[116] Lorenzen J, Buchert R, Bohuslavizki KH. Value of FDG PET in patients with fever of unknown origin. Nucl Med Commun 2001;22:779–83.

[117] Bleeker-Rovers CP, de Kleijn EM, Corstens FH, et al. Clinical value of FDG PET in patients with fever of unknown origin and patients suspected of focal infection or inflammation. Eur J Nucl Med Mol Imaging 2004;31:29–37.

[118] Buysschaert I, Vanderschueren S, Blockmans D, et al. Contribution of (18)fluoro-deoxyglucose positron emission tomography to the work-up of patients with fever of unknown origin. Eur J Intern Med 2004;15:151–6.

[119] Kjaer A, Lebech AM, Eigtved A, et al. Fever of unknown origin: prospective comparison of diagnostic value of 18F-FDG PET and 111In-granulocyte scintigraphy. Eur J Nucl Med Mol Imaging 2004;31:622–6.

POSITRON
EMISSION
TOMOGRAPHY

PET Clin 1 (2006) 179–189

ELSEVIER
SAUNDERS

[18F]Fluorodeoxyglucose PET in Large Vessel Vasculitis

Martin A. Walter, MD

- Giant cell arteritis
- Takayasu's arteritis
- Diagnostic workup in large vessel vasculitis
- [18F]fluorodeoxyglucose PET
- [18F]fluorodeoxyglucose PET scanning protocols for large vessel vasculitis
- [18F]fluorodeoxyglucose PET and atherosclerosis
- [18F]fluorodeoxyglucose PET for diagnosing giant cell arteritis
- [18F]fluorodeoxyglucose PET for diagnosing Takayasu's arteritis
- [18F]fluorodeoxyglucose PET CT in large vessel vasculitis
- Summary
- Acknowledgments
- References

[18F]fluorodeoxyglucose (FDG) PET is a noninvasive metabolic imaging modality based on the regional distribution of [18F]FDG and has become increasingly important in the management of oncologic patients [1]. Remarkable images of patients with active vasculitis have been generated through [18F]FDG-PET scans [2–10]. These images indicate the potential of this technique and imply that [18F] FDG-PET may soon be useful in evaluating patients with several forms of vasculitis, especially large vessel vasculitis.

The family of vasculitides has been defined with reference to the size of vessels involved in large, medium, and small vessel vasculitis [Table 1]. The group of large vessel vasculitides includes giant cell arteritis and Takayasu's arteritis. Both of these diseases are challenging with respect to their diagnosis and follow-up, because affected patients regularly present with a set of nonspecific symptoms and laboratory test results. Consequently, a delayed or even unsuccessful diagnostic workup occurs in several patients. The use of whole-body scanning via

[18F]FDG-PET might facilitate a sensitive metabolic imaging modality that could lead to a shorter and more successful diagnostic workup in the near future.

The current data on [18F]FDG-PET in large vessel vasculitis are still sparse, however. The results of only 12 clinical trials are currently available [Table 2]. In addition, there are no standardized guidelines existing for the indication, performance, interpretation, and description of [18F]FDG-PET in large vessel vasculitis. Therefore, the purpose of this review is to summarize current information on the present clinical data and to assist nuclear medicine and rheumatology practitioners in recommending, performing, and interpreting the results of [18F]FDG-PET in patients with suspected large vessel vasculitis.

Giant cell arteritis

Giant cell arteritis is a granulomatous vasculitis of large- and medium-sized arteries that was first described by Hutchinson [11] in 1890. It usually

Institute of Nuclear Medicine, University Hospital, Petersgraben 4, Basel CH-4031, Switzerland
E-mail address: m.a.walter@gmx.net

doi:10.1016/j.cpet.2006.02.001

Table 1: Classification of vasculitis

Size of vessels	Type of vasculitis	Classification criteria[a]
Large	Giant cell arteritis	Age at onset of disease ≥50 years New headache Temporal artery abnormality Elevated erythrocyte sedimentation rate Abnormal findings on biopsy of temporal artery
	Takayasu's arteritis	Age at onset of disease ≤40 years Claudication of an extremity Decreased brachial artery pulse Difference in systolic blood pressure between arms Bruit over the subclavian arteries or the aorta Narrowing or occlusion of the entire aorta at angiography
Medium	Periarteritis nodosa Kawasaki's arteritis Primary central nervous system vasculitis Buerger's disease	
Small	Wegener's disease Churg-Strauss syndrome Microscopic polyangiitis Henoch-Schönlein purpura Essential cryoglobulinemic vasculitis Cutaneous leukocytoclastic angiitis	

[a] Diagnosis of giant cell arteritis: at least three of five criteria: sensitivity of 93.5%, specificity of 90.5%. Diagnosis of Takayasu's arteritis: at least three of six criteria: sensitivity of 91.2%, specificity of 97.8%.

affects the cranial branches of the arteries originating from the aortic arch, particularly the superficial temporal artery; nevertheless, involvement of the entire aorta and its main branches occurs in approximately 15% of cases [12]. Giant cell arteritis commonly occurs in the white population, with an incidence of approximately 18 per 100,000 persons in the population aged older than 50 years [13–15]; however, autopsy studies suggest that it may be more common than is clinically apparent [16]. It

Table 2: Clinical studies on PET in the detection of large vessel inflammation: the present literature

Authors	Year	Takayasu's arteritis	Giant cell arteritis	Follow-up scans	Reference
Blockmans et al	1999	—	11[a]	—	[62]
Blockmans et al	2000	—	25[a]	—	[63]
Belhocine et al	2002	—	3	3	[64]
Meller et al	2003	5	—	—	[51]
Meller et al	2003	1	14	7	[47]
Bleeker-Rovers et al	2003	1	7[a]	1	[44]
Webb et al	2004	18	—	8	[43]
Brodman et al	2004	—	22	—	[45]
Moosig et al	2004	—	12[a]	8	[46]
Andrews et al	2004	6	—	6	[42]
Scheel et al	2004	—	8	8	[52]
Kobayashi et al	2005	14	—	7	[49]
Walter et al	2005	6	20	4	[48]
Total		51	122	52	

[a] Patients with giant cell arteritis and polymyalgia rheumatica.

rarely occurs in Asians and blacks, and women are affected twice as often as men [13]. Until now, the etiology of giant cell arteritis has remained unknown. The classic histologic picture is granulomatous inflammation in which giant cells are usually located at the connection between the intima and media. Panarteritides with mixed-cell inflammatory infiltrates of lymphomononuclear cells, with occasional neutrophils and eosinophils but without giant cells, are also found [17]. The focal arteritic lesions cause ischemia and subsequently lead to a variety of systemic manifestations, whereas the onset of symptoms may be sudden or gradual. Systemic symptoms are present in most patients [18,19]; among these, headache is probably the most frequent symptom and occurs in two thirds of patients [19]. The symptoms also include myalgia, neck pain, scalp tenderness, jaw claudication, fever, abnormal temporal arteries, polyneuropathy of the arms and legs, transient ischemic attacks, general malaise, fatigue, anorexia, weight loss, depression, and night sweats [18,20,21].

Takayasu's arteritis

Takayasu's arteritis is a large vessel vasculitis that primarily affects the aorta and its main branches as well as the coronary and pulmonary arteries. It is named for Mikito Takayasu, who reported the peculiar wreath-like arteriovenous anastomoses around the papillae in a young woman with pulseless disease in 1908 [22]. The incidence of the disease is approximately 2 per 1,000,000 population, with a mean age at onset of 35 years [23–25] and a prevalence in women approximately 10 times higher than in men. Takayasu's arteritis has a worldwide distribution, although it is considered to be more common in the Orient [26]. Its etiology remains unresolved, and its clinical course includes an early and late phase. Pathology studies in the early phase reveal granulomatous or diffuse productive inflammation in the media and adventitia, with secondary thickening of the intima and occasional perivascular inflammation [27]. Commonly, clinical findings include fever of unknown origin with nonspecific systemic symptoms. Conversely, pathology studies in the late phase show marked thinning of the media, with disruption of elastic fibers, fibrotic thickening of the adventitia, and marked intimal proliferation [27]. Variable ischemic symptoms secondary to arterial stenosis or occlusion or arterial dilatation and aneurysmal formation cause various clinical morbid conditions, such as arm claudication, decreased artery pulses, carotodynia, visual loss, stroke, aortic regurgitation, and hypertension [28]. The topologic classification of Takayasu's arteritis is based on angiographic findings [29], with involvement of branches of the aortic arch (type I); the ascending aorta and the aortic arch and its branches (type IIa); the ascending aorta, the aortic arch and its branches, and the thoracic descending aorta (type IIb); the thoracic descending aorta, the abdominal aorta, or renal arteries (type III); the abdominal aorta or renal arteries (type IV); or combined features of types IIb and IV.

Diagnostic workup in large vessel vasculitis

Giant cell arteritis and Takayasu's arteritis usually present with a wide clinical spectrum; except for the histopathologic findings, there are no laboratory findings specific for either disease. A set of clinical, radiologic, and histologic criteria has been established by the American College of Rheumatology to classify cases of biopsy-proven arteritis [see Table 1] [30,31]. The presence of at least three criteria is required for classifying a patient as having Takayasu's arteritis or giant cell arteritis. These criteria provide a sensitivity of 93.5% with a specificity of 90.5% for diagnosing giant cell arteritis and a sensitivity of 91.2% with a specificity of 97.8% for diagnosing Takayasu's arteritis in biopsy-positive patients. Importantly, the criteria were originally designed for research purposes to help distinguish different types of vasculitis; yet, they are of no use for making the diagnosis in individual patients [32].

This is at least partially attributable to the fact that frequent symptoms of giant cell arteritis, such as jaw claudication, diplopia, neck pain, and elevated C-reactive protein, were not included in the criteria. In contrast, included criteria, such as headache and scalp tenderness, can be attributable to various other diseases. A normal erythrocyte sedimentation rate does not rule out giant cell arteritis, as has been found in up to 30% of patients with biopsy-proven giant cell arteritis [33,34]. Approximately 40% of the patients with giant cell arteritis present with nonspecific symptomatology that does not apply to any set of criteria. Especially in older patients, systemic giant cell arteritis symptoms like fever, anorexia, weight loss, and malaise may focus the diagnostic workup toward a suspected malignancy [35].

Frequent clinical features of Takayasu's arteritis, such as fever, postural dizziness, arthralgias, weight loss, headache, hypertension, elevated erythrocyte sedimentation rate, and anemia, were not included in the classification criteria of the American College of Rheumatology. Conversely, angiographic findings as well as different blood pressure in each arm are part of the diagnostic criteria; however, false-negative angiograms are frequently found in early vasculitis [36,37], and patients with Takayasu's arteritis restricted to the abdominal aorta or its branches or to the pulmonary artery do not have different blood pressure in each arm.

The wide clinical spectrum and diagnostic limitations frequently cause a delay in diagnosis and subsequent treatment of giant cell arteritis and Takayasu's arteritis. The use of [18F]FDG-PET can possibly increase the diagnostic certainty and speed up the detection of disease activity.

[18F]fluorodeoxyglucose PET

[18F]FDG-PET is an operator-independent noninvasive imaging modality based on the regional distribution of [18F]FDG. Deoxyglucose can be labeled with the positron-emitting radionuclide 18fluor and is administered intravenously to patients after fasting. [18F]FDG initially distributes in proportion to the perfusion of the organs, whereby it follows the same uptake metabolic route as glucose. Although [18F]FDG is phosphorylated to [18F]FDG-6-phosphate, it is not further metabolized. By this mechanism and also because of its low membrane permeability, it becomes trapped and is accumulated within the cells. The emitted positron can be detected by a scanner, and a bright signal in the [18F]FDG-PET scan reflects increased glucose metabolism.

Many malignancies have heightened glucose metabolism, and for several years, this property has allowed functional examination with [18F]FDG-PET, especially for staging and follow-up in various types of cancers [1]. Activated inflammatory cells have also been shown to overexpress glucose transporters and accumulate increased amounts of glucose and structurally related substances, such as [18F]FDG [38,39], which provides an important rationale for the use of [18F]FDG-PET in vasculitis.

[18F]fluorodeoxyglucose PET scanning protocols for large vessel vasculitis

The American Association of Nuclear Medicine and the European Association of Nuclear Medicine have established procedure guidelines for tumor imaging with [18F]FDG-PET [40,41]. The guidelines of the American Association of Nuclear Medicine from 1998 recommend fasting for at least 4 hours before the scan. Low blood glucose levels are recommended, the injected [18F]FDG activity should be 350 to 750 MBq, and the acquisition should be started 30 to 40 minutes after injection. In contrast,

the guidelines of the European Association of Nuclear Medicine from 2003 advocate fasting for at least 6 hours before the scan. The blood glucose level should not exceed 130 mg/dL, the injected [18F]FDG activity should be 6 MBq/kg, and acquisition should be started 60 minutes after injection. Guidelines for PET imaging of inflammation, however, are not established by either of these two associations.

Consequently, the present studies [see Table 2] used several different protocols. Prescan fasting intervals of 4 hours [42,43] and 6 hours [44–46] were used. Overnight fasting [47–49] was also utilized. Regarding the applied [18F]FDG dose, body weight–adapted protocols with [18F]FDG at a rate of 5 [48], 6 [49], or 6.5 MBq [45,50] per kilogram of body weight were used, but fixed doses of 296 [51], 370 [47] and 450 [46] MBq were also used. One group routinely administered additional furosemide [44] to accelerate renal [18F]FDG elimination. Most studies on [18F]FDG-PET in large vessel vasculitis did not restrict scanning by maximal glucose levels. Only three studies tolerated maximum serum glucose levels of 100 mg/dL [47,51] and 180 mg/dL [48], respectively. Also, the time interval between [18F]FDG application and image acquisition showed large differences: 45 [48,49], 60 [44,45,47,50,51], and 90 [42,43,46] minutes of [18F]FDG uptake are reported. Generally, dedicated PET scanners with full-ring detectors were used; nevertheless, hybrid cameras have also been successfully employed [47,51,52]. Recently, reports on the use of combined [18F]FDG-PET-CT scanners in large vessel vasculitis have become available [49,53,54].

This summary indicates the present lack of standardization; however, it also demonstrates that [18F]FDG-PET can stably image large vessel vasculitis under a variety of protocols.

[18F]fluorodeoxyglucose PET and atherosclerosis

Not only vasculitic vessels but atherosclerotic plaques have been shown to accumulate glucose analogues [Fig. 1] [55]. As a result, modest large vessel [18F]FDG accumulation at the level of the major vessels occurs in approximately 50% of all PET scans, with increased prevalence in older people [56,57]. This vascular uptake might be explained by smooth muscle metabolism in the media, subendothelial smooth muscle proliferation from senescence, and the presence of macrophages within the atherosclerotic plaque. Thus, vascular uptake found in the [18F]FDG-PET scan is not specific for vasculitis.

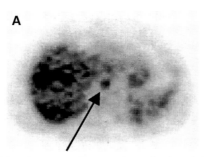
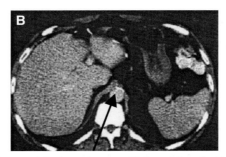

Fig. 1. Axial [18F]FDG-PET images through the abdomen (*A*) show intense FDG activity distributed in the abdominal aorta, whereas the corresponding nonenhanced CT images through the same region (*B*) show the calcified atherosclerotic plaques of the aorta. (*From* Yun M, Yeh D, Araujo LI, et al. F-18 FDG uptake in the large arteries: a new observation. Clin Nucl Med 2001;26(4):314–9; with permission.)

Nonetheless, atherosclerotic lesions can be differentiated from vasculitic lesions by taking into account the vascular distribution, the [^{18}F]FDG uptake pattern, and the intensity of [^{18}F]FDG accumulation. For example, the internal carotid artery demonstrates atherosclerotic changes more frequently, whereas the external carotid artery more often reveals inflammatory changes. The uptake pattern of atherosclerotic mediastinal great vessels sometimes can be identified as ring-shaped structures. Conversely, the uptake pattern in the arteries of the abdomen and lower extremities is often linear and continuous [56]. Most discriminatingly, atherosclerotic lesions rarely demonstrate intense uptake of FDG [47,48].

Accordingly, to differentiate vasculitis from atherosclerosis, visual scoring of vascular [^{18}F]FDG uptake compared with [^{18}F]FDG accumulation in the liver has been established. Accordingly, 3 grades of large vessel [^{18}F]FDG uptake are differentiated [Fig. 2]: grade I, uptake present but lower than liver uptake; grade II, similar to liver uptake; and grade III, uptake higher than liver uptake. This scale was proposed by Meller and colleagues [47] and was subsequently validated to represent the severity of inflammation [48].

So far, this score has been used in two reference patient populations without clinical symptoms or laboratory signs of large vessel inflammation to determine the uptake in nonvasculitic vessels [47,48]. Thereby, grade I vessel uptake was frequently found in the thoracic part of the aorta, which was most likely attributable to atherosclerosis. Accordingly, only grade II or III [^{18}F]FDG uptake in the thoracic aorta and any visible uptake in other segments should routinely be judged as active large vessel inflammation. In this manner, most lesions can be ruled out as being caused by atherosclerosis. Conversely, computed quantification of [^{18}F]FDG uptake by standard uptake value (SUV) has not been shown to be useful in discriminating atherosclerosis from vasculitis to date.

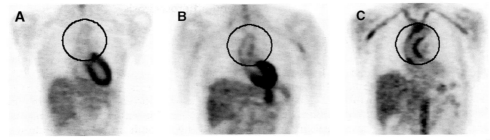

Fig. 2. The visual arteritis score as proposed by Meller and colleagues [47]. The severity of large vessel [^{18}F]FDG uptake is visually graded: grade 1, uptake present but lower than liver uptake (*A*); grade 2, similar to liver uptake (*B*); and grade 3, uptake higher than liver uptake (*C*). (*From* Walter MA, Melzer RA, Schindler C, et al. The value of [18F]FDG-PET in the diagnosis of large-vessel vasculitis and the assessment of activity and extent of disease. Eur J Nucl Med Mol Imaging 2005;32(6):676; with permission.)

[^{18}F]fluorodeoxyglucose PET for diagnosing giant cell arteritis

Today, the diagnosis of giant cell arteritis is mainly based on clinical evaluation, laboratory results, and temporal biopsy. In addition, no imaging modality has been included in the American College of Rheumatology diagnostic criteria for giant cell arteritis [see Table 1]. Nevertheless, [^{18}F]FDG-PET has indicated its usefulness in a number of studies with better evidence as compared with Takayasu's arteritis because of the higher frequency of the disease. Currently, the reports on nine studies including 118 patients are available on use of [^{18}F]FDG-PET in giant cell arteritis [see Table 2].

The common uptake pattern found in great vessels affected by giant cell arteritis was linear and continuous, and the predominant uptake was grade II. Overall, thoracic vessels were most frequently affected, followed by abdominal vessels [47,48]. The ability to detect large vessel inflammation differed considerably in the available publications. In studies using patient populations with polymyalgia rheumatica and giant cell arteritis, patient sensitivities between 56% and 100% were reported [44,45, 50,52], with a specificity between 77% and 98% [50]. These differences can partially be explained by the inclusion of patients with dissimilar activity of the disease. Accordingly, a recent study could confirm that high sensitivities are achieved, especially in the state of active inflammation [Fig. 3]. Thereby, the C-reactive protein has been shown to

be a better predictor for the sensitivity of [^{18}F]FDG-PET in giant cell arteritis than the erythrocyte sedimentation rate [48].

Comparative studies using [^{18}F]FDG-PET and MRI revealed comparable sensitivities of the two methods, but [^{18}F]FDG-PET has been shown to identify significantly more affected vascular regions [47,52]. These results reflect the advantage of metabolic imaging, because metabolic changes normally precede morphologic changes in giant cell arteritis. Moreover, [^{18}F]FDG-PET might also allow new insights into the pathologic findings of giant cell arteritis and polymyalgia rheumatica. A study in patients with polymyalgia rheumatica demonstrated inflammation of the aorta or its major branches in 92% of patients. The tracer uptake was strongly correlated to the erythrocyte sedimentation rate and the C-reactive protein. These data indicate that polymyalgia rheumatica is frequently accompanied by subclinical vasculitis [46].

Moreover, [^{18}F]FDG-PET offers the possibility of whole-body screening in one procedure. Thus, it might become helpful in the follow-up of patients with giant cell arteritis. [^{18}F]FDG-PET results have shown good correlation with the clinical course, which was also confirmed by computed quantification of the vascular [^{18}F]FDG accumulation [46]. Compared with the MRI results, the follow-up results of [^{18}F]FDG-PET correlate significantly better with clinical improvement [47], because [^{18}F]FDG-PET is able to monitor changes in metabolic activity directly.

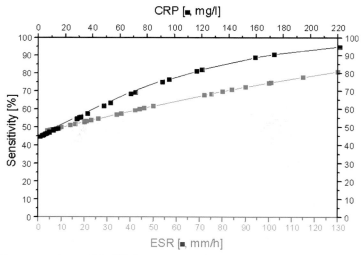

Fig. 3. Sensitivity of large vessel vasculitis. [^{18}F]FDG-PET uptake as a function of the C-reactive protein (CRP) and erythrocyte sedimentation rate (ESR) levels, respectively. High sensitivity for detection of large vessel vasculitis is reached at high CRP and ESR levels. (*From* Walter MA, Melzer RA, Schindler C, et al. The value of [18F]FDG-PET in the diagnosis of large-vessel vasculitis and the assessment of activity and extent of disease. Eur J Nucl Med Mol Imaging 2005;32(6):677; with permission.)

The value of [^{18}F]FDG-PET for diagnosing temporal arteritis has recently been investigated in a study comprising 22 patients [45]. Of these patients, 17 had involvement of the temporal arteries; however, no such involvement was detected by [^{18}F]FDG-PET. This limitation of [^{18}F]FDG-PET is mainly attributable to the high [^{18}F]FDG uptake in the brain and the small diameter of the temporal arteries. Thus, direct evaluation of the temporal arteries does not seem to be feasible with current whole-body PET techniques.

[^{18}F]fluorodeoxyglucose PET for diagnosing Takayasu's arteritis

In contrast to giant cell arteritis, the initial diagnosis of Takayasu's arteritis is partly based on morphologic imaging. The results of angiography are also integrated in the diagnostic criteria of the American College of Rheumatology [see Table 2]. Angiographic alterations usually occur in the late phase of Takayasu's arteritis, however, and metabolic imaging with [^{18}F]FDG-PET facilitates detection of metabolic changes during the early phase. To date, the data on the use of [^{18}F]FDG-PET in Takayasu's arteritis are poor compared with the data on [^{18}F]FDG-PET in giant cell arteritis because of the rarity of the disease. Only seven studies including a total of 51 patients have been reported on to date.

The common [^{18}F]FDG uptake pattern in the early phase of Takayasu's arteritis is linear and continuous [Fig. 4A], whereas in the late phase, it can become patchy rather than continuous but still in a linear distribution [43]. Based on the present data, the diagnostic value of [^{18}F]FDG-PET seems to be consistently high in Takayasu's arteritis. Two studies reported sensitivities of 83% and 100% [42,51], whereas another report found a sensitivity of 92%, with a specificity of 100% and a diagnostic accuracy of 94% [43]. These sensitivities are comparable to those of MRI; however, metabolic imaging using [^{18}F]FDG-PET in Takayasu's arteritis has been shown to identify more affected vascular regions than morphologic imaging with MRI [51]. Nevertheless, it has to be mentioned that [^{18}F]FDG-PET does not provide any information about changes in the wall structure or luminal blood flow.

Similar to the situation in giant cell arteritis, there is a clear correlation between the activity of large vessel inflammation and the ability of [^{18}F]FDG-PET to detect inflammatory vessels. In a recent study, [^{18}F]FDG-PET–positive patients showed significantly higher erythrocyte sedimentation rates and C-reactive protein levels as compared with [^{18}F]FDG-PET–negative patients, with the C-reactive protein as a superior marker [43].

A follow-up in Takayasu's arteritis only based on clinical symptoms has been shown to be rather limited. In a previous report, biopsy demonstrated active inflammation in 44% of patients thought to be in clinical remission [58]. Conversely, [^{18}F]FDG-PET is able to detect more sites than just those that were clinically active [43]. Because of its high sensitivity and the good correlation with outcome,

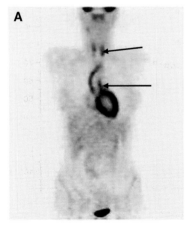
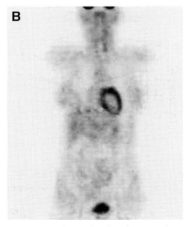

Fig. 4. (*A*) [^{18}F]FDG-PET scan of a patient with Takayasu's arteritis, with markedly abnormal uptake of [^{18}F]FDG in the aortic arch and carotid arteries (*arrows*). (*B*) [^{18}F]FDG-PET scan of the same patient in clinical remission after treatment with prednisone and intravenous cyclophosphamide. (*From* Andrews J, Al-Nahhas A, Pennell DJ, et al. Non-invasive imaging in the diagnosis and management of Takayasu's arteritis. Ann Rheum Dis 2004;63(8):998; with permission.)

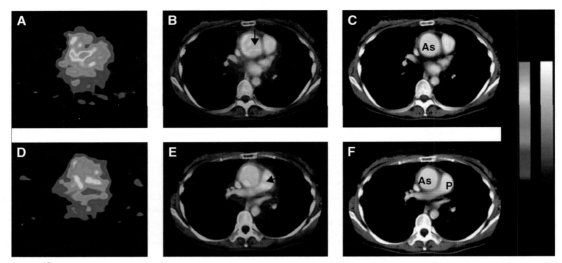

Fig. 5. [^{18}F]FDG-PET scan coregistered with enhanced CT scan of a patient with active Takayasu's arteritis revealed that [^{18}F]FDG accumulations were localized in the vascular wall of the ascending aortic and pulmonary artery. (*A, D*) Axial images of the [^{18}F]FDG-PET with [^{18}F]FDG accumulation in the mediastinum. Coregistered PET scan with enhanced CT images. The arrows indicate [^{18}F]FDG accumulation in the ascending aorta (*B*) and pulmonary arteries (*E*). (*C, F*) Enhanced reconstituted CT images of the same level as A and D. The ascending aorta was enlarged, causing aortic regurgitation. As, ascending aorta; P, pulmonary artery. (*From* Kobayashi Y, Ishii K, Oda K, et al. Aortic wall inflammation due to Takayasu arteritis imaged with 18F-FDG PET coregistered with enhanced CT. J Nucl Med 2005;46(6):919; with permission.)

[^{18}F]FDG-PET is a promising candidate to be used regularly in the follow-up of Takayasu's arteritis [see Fig. 4] [42,43,48].

[^{18}F]fluorodeoxyglucose PET CT in large vessel vasculitis

The combination of [^{18}F]FDG-PET scanners with CT scanners is becoming increasingly important in the management of oncologic patients [59–61]. The combination of both techniques allows the integration of morphologic and metabolic information for detection, staging, and therapy control. The rapidly increasing availability of [^{18}F]FDG-PET-CT scanners is also introducing new opportunities for their application in rheumatology. The use of combined [^{18}F]FDG-PET-CT scanners should allow the investigation of the morphology and metabolic activity of affected vessels. Moreover, the localization of affected segments should be significantly improved. Two case reports have already indicated the value of [^{18}F]FDG-PET-CT scanners in large vessel vasculitis [52,53], and one clinical trial has investigated the value of the combination of both modalities in 14 patients [49]. The coregistered CT scan was most useful for the anatomic identification of vascular [^{18}F]FDG uptake, especially in the case of rather moderate [^{18}F]FDG accumulation. Furthermore, the anatomic identification of medi-astinal [^{18}F]FDG uptake, particularly in the pulmonary arteries, was significantly improved [Fig. 5]. The evaluation of [^{18}F]FDG-PET-CT scanners in large vessel vasculitis is ongoing; however, the first results are quite promising.

Summary

In conclusion, whole-body imaging with [^{18}F]FDG-PET is highly effective in assessing the activity and extent of giant cell arteritis and Takayasu's arteritis, respectively:

> Metabolic imaging using [^{18}F]FDG-PET has been shown to identify more affected vascular regions than morphologic imaging with MRI in both diseases.
> The visual grading of vascular [^{18}F]FDG uptake helps to discriminate arteritis from atherosclerosis and therefore provides high specificity.
> High sensitivity is attained by scanning during the active inflammatory phase.

Thus, [^{18}F]FDG-PET has the potential to develop into a valuable tool in the diagnostic workup of giant cell arteritis and Takayasu's arteritis, respectively, and might become a first-line investigation technique. Consensus regarding the most favorable imaging procedure as well as further clinical evidence is urgently needed, however.

Acknowledgments

The author is grateful to Ralf Melzer, Helmut Rasch, and Allan Tyndall for their most helpful comments on the article.

References

[1] Rohren EM, Turkington TG, Coleman RE. Clinical applications of PET in oncology. Radiology 2004;231(2):305–32.

[2] Turlakow A, Yeung HW, Pui J, et al. Fludeoxyglucose positron emission tomography in the diagnosis of giant cell arteritis. Arch Intern Med 2001;161(7):1003–7.

[3] Blockmans D, Van Moer E, Dehem J, et al. Positron emission tomography can reveal abdominal periaortitis. Clin Nucl Med 2002;27(3):211–2.

[4] Wenger M, Gasser R, Donnemiller E, et al. Images in cardiovascular medicine. Generalized large vessel arteritis visualized by 18 fluorodeoxyglucose-positron emission tomography. Circulation 2003;107(6):923.

[5] Brodmann M, Lipp RW, Aigner R, et al. Positron emission tomography reveals extended thoracic and abdominal peri-aortitis. Vasc Med 2003; 8(2):127–8.

[6] Wiest R, Gluck T, Schonberger J, et al. Clinical image: occult large vessel vasculitis diagnosed by PET imaging. Rheumatol Int 2001;20(6):250.

[7] De Winter F, Petrovic M, Van de Wiele C, et al. Imaging of giant cell arteritis: evidence of splenic involvement using FDG positron emission tomography. Clin Nucl Med 2000;25(8):633–4.

[8] Hara M, Goodman PC, Leder RA. FDG-PET finding in early-phase Takayasu arteritis. J Comput Assist Tomogr 1999;23(1):16–8.

[9] Malik IS, Harare O, Al-Nahhas A, et al. Takayasu's arteritis: management of left main stem stenosis. Heart 2003;89(3):e9.

[10] Walter MA, Melzer RA, Graf M, et al. [18F]FDG-PET of giant-cell aortitis. Rheumatology (Oxford) 2005;44(5):690–1.

[11] Hutchinson J. On a peculiar form of thrombotic arteritis of the aged which is sometimes productive or gangrene. Arch Surg 1890;1:323–9.

[12] Klein RG, Hunder GG, Stanson AW, et al. Large artery involvement in giant cell (temporal) arteritis. Ann Intern Med 1975;83(6):806–12.

[13] Salvarani C, Gabriel SE, O'Fallon WM, et al. The incidence of giant cell arteritis in Olmsted County, Minnesota: apparent fluctuations in a cyclic pattern. Ann Intern Med 1995;123(3): 192–4.

[14] Franzen P, Sutinen S, von Knorring J. Giant cell arteritis and polymyalgia rheumatica in a region of Finland: an epidemiologic, clinical and pathologic study, 1984–1988. J Rheumatol 1992; 19(2):273–6.

[15] Gonzalez-Gay MA, Alonso MD, Aguero JJ, et al. Giant cell arteritis in Mediterranean countries: comment on the article by Salvarani et al. Arthritis Rheum 1992;35(10):1249–50.

[16] Ostberg G. An arteritis with special reference to polymyalgia arteritica. Acta Pathol Microbiol Scand [A] 1973;237(Suppl 237):1–59.

[17] Lie JT. Illustrated histopathologic classification criteria for selected vasculitis syndromes. American College of Rheumatology Subcommittee on Classification of Vasculitis. Arthritis Rheum 1990;33(8):1074–87.

[18] Weyand CM. The Dunlop-Dottridge Lecture: the pathogenesis of giant cell arteritis. J Rheumatol 2000;27(2):517–22.

[19] Salvarani C, Macchioni PL, Tartoni PL, et al. Polymyalgia rheumatica and giant cell arteritis: a 5-year epidemiologic and clinical study in Reggio Emilia, Italy. Clin Exp Rheumatol 1987; 5(3):205–15.

[20] Huston KA, Hunder GG. Giant cell (cranial) arteritis: a clinical review. Am Heart J 1980;100(1): 99–105.

[21] Calamia KT, Hunder GG. Giant cell arteritis (temporal arteritis) presenting as fever of undetermined origin. Arthritis Rheum 1981;24(11):1414–8.

[22] Takayasu M. Case with unusual changes of the central vessels in the retina. Acta Soc Ophthal Jpn 1908;12:554–5.

[23] Waern AU, Andersson P, Hemmingsson A. Takayasu's arteritis: a hospital-region based study on occurrence, treatment and prognosis. Angiology 1983;34(5):311–20.

[24] Hall S, Barr W, Lie JT, et al. Takayasu arteritis. A study of 32 North American patients. Medicine (Baltimore) 1985;64(2):89–99.

[25] el-Reshaid K, Varro J, al-Duwairi Q, et al. Takayasu's arteritis in Kuwait. J Trop Med Hyg 1995;98(5):299–305.

[26] Lande A. Abdominal Takayasu's aortitis, the middle aortic syndrome and atherosclerosis. A critical review. Int Angiol 1998;17(1):1–9.

[27] Nasu T. Pathology of pulseless disease. A systematic study and critical review of twenty-one autopsy cases reported in Japan. Angiology 1963; 14:225–42.

[28] Matsunaga N, Hayashi K, Sakamoto I, et al. Takayasu arteritis: protean radiologic manifestations and diagnosis. Radiographics 1997;17(3): 579–94.

[29] Moriwaki R, Noda M, Yajima M, et al. Clinical manifestations of Takayasu arteritis in India and Japan: new classification of angiographic findings. Angiology 1997;48(5):369–79.

[30] Hunder GG, Bloch DA, Michel BA, et al. The American College of Rheumatology 1990 criteria for the classification of giant cell arteritis. Arthritis Rheum 1990;33(8):1122–8.

[31] Arend WP, Michel BA, Bloch DA, et al. The American College of Rheumatology 1990 criteria for the classification of Takayasu arteritis. Arthritis Rheum 1990;33(8):1129–34.

[32] Rao JK, Allen NB, Pincus T. Limitations of the 1990 American College of Rheumatology classi-

fication criteria in the diagnosis of vasculitis. Ann Intern Med 1998;129(5):345–52.

[33] Salvarani C, Hunder GG. Giant cell arteritis with low erythrocyte sedimentation rate: frequency of occurrence in a population-based study. Arthritis Rheum 2001;45(2):140–5.

[34] Hayreh SS, Zimmerman B. Management of giant cell arteritis. Our 27-year clinical study: new light on old controversies. Ophthalmologica 2003; 217(4):239–59.

[35] Gonzalez-Gay MA, Garcia-Porrua C, Salvarani C, et al. The spectrum of conditions mimicking polymyalgia rheumatica in Northwestern Spain. J Rheumatol 2000;27(9):2179–84.

[36] Lambert M, Hachulla E, Hatron PY, et al. [Takayasu's arteritis: vascular investigations and therapeutic management. Experience with 16 patients]. Rev Med Interne 1998;19(12):878–84. [in French].

[37] Lambert M, Hatron PY, Hachulla E, et al. Takayasu's arteritis diagnosed at the early systemic phase: diagnosis with noninvasive investigation despite normal findings on angiography. J Rheumatol 1998;25(2):376–7.

[38] Ishimori T, Saga T, Mamede M, et al. Increased (18)F-FDG uptake in a model of inflammation: concanavalin A-mediated lymphocyte activation. J Nucl Med 2002;43(5):658–63.

[39] Jones HA, Cadwallader KA, White JF, et al. Dissociation between respiratory burst activity and deoxyglucose uptake in human neutrophil granulocytes: implications for interpretation of (18)F-FDG PET images. J Nucl Med 2002;43(5): 652–7.

[40] Schelbert HR, Hoh CK, Royal HD, et al. Procedure guideline for tumor imaging using fluorine-18-FDG. Society of Nuclear Medicine. J Nucl Med 1998;39(7):1302–5.

[41] Bombardieri E, Aktolun C, Baum RP, et al. FDG-PET: procedure guidelines for tumour imaging. Eur J Nucl Med Mol Imaging 2003;30(12): BP115–24.

[42] Andrews J, Al-Nahhas A, Pennell DJ, et al. Noninvasive imaging in the diagnosis and management of Takayasu's arteritis. Ann Rheum Dis 2004;63(8):995–1000.

[43] Webb M, Chambers A, Al-Nahhas A, et al. The role of 18F-FDG PET in characterising disease activity in Takayasu arteritis. Eur J Nucl Med Mol Imaging 2004;31(5):627–34.

[44] Bleeker-Rovers CP, Bredie SJ, van der Meer JW, et al. F-18-fluorodeoxyglucose positron emission tomography in diagnosis and follow-up of patients with different types of vasculitis. Neth J Med 2003;61(10):323–9.

[45] Brodmann M, Lipp RW, Passath A, et al. The role of 2-18F-fluoro-2-deoxy-D-glucose positron emission tomography in the diagnosis of giant cell arteritis of the temporal arteries. Rheumatology (Oxford) 2004;43(2):241–2.

[46] Moosig F, Czech N, Mehl C, et al. Correlation between 18-fluorodeoxyglucose accumulation in large vessels and serological markers of inflammation in polymyalgia rheumatica: a quantitative PET study. Ann Rheum Dis 2004;63(7): 870–3.

[47] Meller J, Strutz F, Siefker U, et al. Early diagnosis and follow-up of aortitis with [(18)F]FDG PET and MRI. Eur J Nucl Med Mol Imaging 2003; 30(5):730–6.

[48] Walter MA, Melzer RA, Schindler C, et al. The value of [18F]FDG-PET in the diagnosis of large-vessel vasculitis and the assessment of activity and extent of disease. Eur J Nucl Med Mol Imaging 2005;32(6):674–81.

[49] Kobayashi Y, Ishii K, Oda K, et al. Aortic wall inflammation due to Takayasu arteritis imaged with 18F-FDG PET coregistered with enhanced CT. J Nucl Med 2005;46(6):917–22.

[50] Blockmans D, Stroobants S, Maes A, et al. Positron emission tomography in giant cell arteritis and polymyalgia rheumatica: evidence for inflammation of the aortic arch. Am J Med 2000; 108(3):246–9.

[51] Meller J, Grabbe E, Becker W, et al. Value of F-18 FDG hybrid camera PET and MRI in early Takayasu aortitis. Eur Radiol 2003;13(2):400–5.

[52] Scheel AK, Meller J, Vosshenrich R, et al. Diagnosis and follow up of aortitis in the elderly. Ann Rheum Dis 2004;63(11):1507–10.

[53] Kroger K, Antoch G, Goyen M, et al. Positron emission tomography/computed tomography improves diagnostics of inflammatory arteritis. Heart Vessels 2005;20(4):179–83.

[54] Antoch G, Freudenberg LS, Debatin JF, et al. Images in vascular medicine. Diagnosis of giant cell arteritis with PET/CT. Vasc Med 2003;8(4): 281–2.

[55] Rudd JH, Warburton EA, Fryer TD, et al. Imaging atherosclerotic plaque inflammation with [18F]-fluorodeoxyglucose positron emission tomography. Circulation 2002;105(23):2708–11.

[56] Yun M, Yeh D, Araujo LI, et al. F-18 FDG uptake in the large arteries: a new observation. Clin Nucl Med 2001;26(4):314–9.

[57] Yun M, Jang S, Cucchiara A, et al. 18F FDG uptake in the large arteries: a correlation study with the atherogenic risk factors. Semin Nucl Med 2002;32(1):70–6.

[58] Kerr GS, Hallahan CW, Giordano J, et al. Takayasu arteritis. Ann Intern Med 1994;120(11):919–29.

[59] Sachelarie I, Kerr K, Ghesani M, et al. Integrated PET-CT: evidence-based review of oncology indications. Oncology (Williston Park) 2005;19(4): 481–90.

[60] Macapinlac HA. FDG PET and PET/CT imaging in lymphoma and melanoma. Cancer J 2004; 10(4):262–70.

[61] Frank SJ, Chao KS, Schwartz DL, et al. Technology insight: PET and PET/CT in head and neck tumor staging and radiation therapy planning. Nat Clin Pract Oncol 2005;2(10):526–33.

[62] Blockmans D, Maes A, Stroobants S, et al. New arguments for a vasculitic nature of polymyalgia

rheumatica using positron emission tomography. Rheumatology (Oxford) 1999;38(5):444–7.

[63] Blockmans D, Baeyens H, Van Loon R, et al. Peri-aortitis and aortic dissection due to Wegener's granulomatosis. Clin Rheumatol 2000;19(2): 161–4.

[64] Belhocine T, Kaye O, Delanaye P, et al. [Horton's disease and extra-temporal vessel locations: role of 18FDG PET scan. Report of 3 cases and review of the literature]. Rev Med Interne 2002;23(7): 584–91 [in French].

POSITRON
EMISSION
TOMOGRAPHY

PET Clin 1 (2006) 191–198

Assessment of Therapy Response by Fluorine-18 Fluorodeoxyglucose PET in Infection and Inflammation

Rakesh Kumar, MD[a],*, Anil Chauhan, MD[a],
Hongming Zhuang, MD, PhD[b], Abass Alavi, MD[b]

- Overview of PET in infection or inflammation
- Specific inflammatory or infectious lesions
  Vasculitis
  Bone infection

Prosthesis infection
Atherosclerosis
Others
- Summary
- References

Fluorine-18 fluoro-deoxyglucose (FDG) PET has proven particularly helpful in oncology, where its applications include initial diagnosis, staging, and therapeutic follow-up studies [1–3]. Its role is continuously increasing over time because of improvements in technical aspects and the introduction of PET/CT. Being a functional study, FDG-PET assesses the tissue metabolism. In theory, functional imaging has superior sensitivity because it can detect abnormal metabolic function in pathologic lesions before any structural changes become detectable. Whenever a pathologic process begins, there must be an initial metabolic change or reaction on the molecular level that leads to the development of pathologic change. These changes, in turn, lead to the eventual development of gross structural abnormalities through infection, inflammation, or pathologic growth. Consequently, the ability of functional imaging technologies to detect these initial metabolic changes results in the aforementioned higher sensitivity in the detection of pathologic change as compared with structural imaging technologies, which depend on the structural

changes occurring later on. PET shows positive uptake in any tissue in the body with increased metabolism, whether this is a benign, malignant, or even normal physiologic process. This mechanism has been exploited recently to assess the role of PET in benign disorders, especially inflammatory or infectious diseases.

PET is a well-known imaging modality in assessing the treatment response to chemotherapy or radiotherapy in various malignancies [4–6]. Little is known about the role of FDG-PET for assessing the treatment response in inflammatory or infectious diseases, however. A systematic review of the literature reveals few publications reporting evaluation of the treatment response using PET. The clinical value of FDG-PET in the assessment of therapy response is mostly reported in patients with vasculitis. In other infectious diseases, such as osteomyelitis, prosthesis infection, and atherosclerosis, few studies have been described. Nevertheless, if we extrapolate the previously mentioned use of PET in inflammatory or infectious diseases, it may be assumed that PET holds a promising future

[a] Department of Nuclear Medicine, All India Institute of Medical Sciences, New Delhi 110020, India
[b] Division of Nuclear Medicine, Department of Radiology, Hospital of the University of Pennsylvania, Philadelphia, PA 19104, USA
* Corresponding author.
E-mail address: rkphulia@yahoo.com (R. Kumar).

doi:10.1016/j.cpet.2006.03.002

role in the follow-up of inflammatory or infectious diseases.

Overview of PET in infection or inflammation

A PET scan, being a functional imaging modality, is expected to be useful in early detection, delineating the actual lesion, and monitoring the treatment response when compared with conventional imaging, such as CT, MRI, and ultrasonography (USG). Unlike CT, it is safe and noninvasive (no contrast used), and unlike MRI, it can be used in patients with metallic implants. FDG is the most commonly used radiotracer in characterizing inflammatory or infectious lesions. The role of FDG-PET was demonstrated in 1987, when Theron and Tyler [7] reported the usefulness of FDG-PET in the diagnosis and treatment of Takayasu arteritis (TA). In next 1.5 decades, many authors reported the increased uptake of FDG in various infectious or inflammatory lesions.

FDG is a radioactive analogue of glucose and is able to detect altered glucose metabolism in pathologic processes. Various glucose receptors are involved in the uptake of FDG in a cell, as they are in the case of glucose. After entering the cell, FDG is phosphorylated to FDG-6-phosphate by the glycolytic enzyme hexokinase. The next enzyme in glycolysis, glucose-6-phosphate isomerase, does not act on FDG-6-phosphate, however, leading to entrapment of FDG in the cell. It can be concluded that FDG uptake is directly proportional to the level of glycolysis in the cell. Therefore, it can be expected to increase in malignant lesions, certain benign lesions, inflammatory lesions, and infectious lesions as well as normally in organs, such as the brain, heart, and endometrium. The uptake is nonspecific, however, and it can sometimes be difficult to differentiate between benign and malignant lesions as well as between infections and sterile inflammation.

Inflammatory lesions are known to cause misinterpretation of the findings in patients with malignancy, usually arising as postbiopsy inflammation. Several investigators have suggested dual-time-point PET to differentiate between malignancy and inflammation [8–10]. Malignant lesions typically have increased uptake of FDG for several hours before a peak standard uptake value (SUV) is reached, whereas FDG uptake is reduced in inflammatory lesions over time. The results of various reports on breast, lung, and head and neck cancers support these predictions [8–10]. Kumar and colleagues [9] demonstrated an average SUV increase of 12.6% between the two time points in breast cancer. Conversely, inflammation showed a decrease in the average SUV of −10.2% over the time. The au-

thors reported a cutoff value of 3.75 or more in SUV in differentiating inflammatory and malignant lesions. Similarly, in head and neck cancers, Hustinx and coworkers [10] reported an average 23% SUV increase between the two time points. Sites of inflammation had SUV changes that varied from −2.4% to 2.8%, which was significantly less than the SUV changes seen in the malignant lesions. In addition to the early detection of inflammation, the future holds great promise for the role of FDG-PET in the follow-up of patients with inflammatory lesions, whether they are sterile inflammatory lesions or infectious lesions. FDG-PET demonstrates early change as decreased FDG uptake if the inflammatory lesions respond to the treatment. Conversely, it also holds true that FDG-PET shows persistently increased uptake if the inflammatory lesions do not respond to the treatment. This area needs intensive work, but FDG-PET might be a promising imaging modality in future in this regard.

Specific inflammatory or infectious lesions

Vasculitis

Vasculitis is a group of multiple different disorders characterized by pathologic inflammatory features in the blood vessel walls. These disorders are primarily classified on the basis of the size of predominantly involved vessels. In 1987, Theron and Tyler [7] reported on the usefulness of FDG-PET in the diagnosis and treatment of a case of TA. Since then, many authors have supported the role of FDG-PET in patients with vasculitis, especially TA and giant cell arteritis [11–24].

In addition to early diagnosis, another important aspect in the management of vasculitis is detection of the treatment response at the earliest possible point so that early intervention can be instituted appropriately. Many authors have reported on the usefulness of FDG-PET to determine whether or not there is an appropriate response to therapy in the follow-up of patients with vasculitis [Table 1] [7,15–24]. Derdelinckx and colleagues [15] reported the case of a 62-year-old female patient with thoracic aortitis. The primary diagnosis was based on CT, MRI, and FDG-PET scan findings. There was FDG uptake in baseline PET study that returned to normal along with other inflammatory parameters after treatment with corticosteroids. The authors proposed the usefulness of FDG-PET in the early diagnosis and monitoring of the treatment response in this inflammatory aortic disorder. Turlakow and coworkers [16] reported a case of giant cell arteritis, which presented as fever of unknown origin and raised erythrocyte segmentation rate

Table 1: **Fluorine-18 fluorodeoxyglucose PET studies for diagnosis and evaluation of the treatment response in patients with vasculitis**

Study no.	Authors	Year	Type of study	No. patients followed up	Diagnosis
1	Theron and Tyler [7]	1987	Case report	1	TA
2	Derdelinckx et al [15]	2000	Case report	1	Aortitis
3	Turlakow et al [16]	2001	Case report	1	GCA
4	Meller et al [17]	2003	Evaluation study	6	GCA
5	Bleeker-Rovers et al [19]	2003	Evaluation study	5	PAN + GCA + WG
6	de Leeuw et al [21]	2004	Case series	5	GCA + TA
7	Bleeker-Rovers et al [20]	2004	Case reports	3	PAN + WG + GCA
8	Webb et al [22]	2004	Evaluation study	8	TA
9	Andrews et al [23]	2004	Evaluation study	6	TA
10	Scheel et al [24]	2004	Evaluation study	8	Aortitis
11	Moreno et al [18]	2005	Case reports	2	TA

Abbreviations: GCA, giant cell arteritis; PAN, polyarteritis nodosa; TA, Takayasu arteritis; WG, Wegener granulomatosis.

(ESR). A CT scan of chest showed a mediastinal mass suggestive of malignancy. FDG-PET revealed high FDG uptake in the entire aorta; left main coronary artery; and subclavian, carotid, and common iliac arteries bilaterally. A follow-up PET scan obtained after 2 weeks of steroid therapy showed normalization of FDG uptake.

In a prospective study of 15 patients with aortitis, Meller and colleagues [17] compared FDG-PET with MRI for diagnosis and evaluation of the treatment response. A PET scan showed pathologic FDG uptake in 56% (59 of 104) of the vascular regions studied. Of the seven follow-up PET scans performed in 6 patients after starting immunosuppressive medication, 80% (24 of 30) of the vascular regions showing initial pathologic uptake of FDG showed normalization. This normalization of FDG uptake was well correlated with clinical improvement and normalization of the laboratory findings. Of 76 vascular regions studied in 13 patients, 41 (53%) showed vasculitis on MRI. Of 76 vascular regions studied with PET and MRI, 47 were concordantly positive or negative on both modalities, 11 were positive on MRI only, and 18 were positive on PET only. MRI was performed during follow-up in 6 patients: of 17 regions with inflammatory changes, 15 regions remained unchanged and 2 showed improvement. The authors concluded that the results of FDG-PET and MRI were comparable for the diagnosis of aortitis but that FDG imaging identified more vascular regions involved in the inflammatory process than did MRI.

Moreno and coworkers [18] reported two cases of TA showing intense uptake of FDG in PET imaging. The first case showed normalization of FDG uptake on steroid maintenance, which again increased as the steroid dose was decreased and symptoms started again. The second case remained asymptomatic for 4 months; however, as the steroid dose

was decreased from 30 to 20 mg/d, the patient became symptomatic and showed intense FDG uptake on PET. In these two cases, PET was found to be a useful technique for diagnosing TA and showed good correlation with disease activity. Bleeker-Rovers and colleagues [19] evaluated the role of FDG-PET in 20 patients with suspected vasculitis, 2 patients with fever of unknown origin, and 5 patients for follow-up of vasculitis. All 5 patients who came for follow-up demonstrated a good clinical and biochemical response to the therapy. In all these patients, FDG uptake returned to normal levels when compared with baseline FDG uptake. In another study, Bleeker-Rovers and colleagues [20] reported three cases with vasculitis (one with polyarteritis nodosa, one with Wegener granulomatosis, and one with giant cell arteritis). All 3 patients initially showed increased FDG uptake on the baseline FDG-PET scan, which was normalized after steroid therapy. There was good correlation of FDG uptake and disease activity in all 3 patients. de Leeuw and coworkers [21] assessed FDG-PET in the diagnosis and follow-up of TA and giant cell arteritis in 5 consecutive patients and compared it with angiography, magnetic resonance angiography (MRA), and clinical parameters. FDG-PET was able to visualize inflamed arteries in all 5 patients, but there was a discrepancy between PET and angiography or MRA. After treatment and the disappearance of clinical symptoms, FDG uptake was clearly reduced compared with that shown in the baseline scan in all patients. Webb and colleagues [22] evaluated the role of FDG-PET by reviewing 28 scans performed in 18 patients suspected of having TA. FDG-PET had a sensitivity, specificity, positive predictive value (PPV), and negative predictive value (NPV) of 92%, 100%, 85%, and 100%, respectively, in the initial assessment of active vasculitis in TA. There were 10 follow-up FDG-PET scans in 8 of 18 patients, and all showed universal agreement with the clinical assessment of disease activity scores.

Andrews and coworkers [23] evaluated FDG-PET and MRI for diagnosis and therapy response in six patients with TA. Five of six patients demonstrated remission on appropriate treatment clinically and biochemically. In these five patients, FDG uptake returned to normal levels after treatment. In one patient, who had active disease on follow-up, FDG-PET showed persistently increased FDG uptake. Follow-up MRI was performed in five of six patients and showed resolution of wall thickening only in one patient and no progression of the disease in four patients. Scheel and colleagues [24] evaluated the correlation of MRI and FDG-PET with the clinical course and inflammatory markers in eight patients with aortitis. At diagnosis, 20 of 24 vascular regions from eight patients were positive by FDG-PET scan and 15 of 21 aortic regions were positive by MRI. Patients were treated with corticosteroids. By FDG-PET scan, 11 (55%) of 20 pathologic aortic regions returned to normal in the follow-up examination, which correlated closely with the clinical and laboratory follow-up examination. Conversely, by MRI, 14 of 15 initially affected vascular regions were unchanged. The authors concluded that FDG-PET and MRI are both effective techniques for detecting early aortitis and have a high correlation with laboratory inflammatory measures. Nevertheless, FDG-PET is a better modality as compared with MRI in evaluating therapy response during the follow-up examination. A decrease in FDG uptake was well correlated with the clinical symptoms and inflammatory serum markers.

After reviewing the literature, it is clear that FDG-PET has a definite role in the establishment of a diagnosis, in the acquisition of knowledge regarding the extent of the disease, and in evaluation of the treatment response and disease activity in patients with vasculitis. In three studies, which involved 20 patients with vasculitis who underwent baseline and follow-up study, FDG-PET was compared with MRI for diagnosis and evaluation of the therapy response [17,23,24]. All these studies demonstrated that FDG-PET and MRI are both effective noninvasive techniques for detecting early aortitis. FDG-PET was better than MRI in demonstrating normalization of disease activity after treatment during the follow-up examination, however.

Bone infection

Bone infections can be acute or chronic. Diagnosis is usually made on clinical grounds and is aided by biochemical parameters, plain radiographs, bone scintigraphy, and MRI. In bone infections, FDG-

PET has been investigated for acute and chronic osteomyelitis [25–29]. Kalicke and coworkers [28] evaluated the role of FDG-PET in acute and chronic osteomyelitis and inflammatory spondylitis. They analyzed 15 patients who underwent surgery after bone infection and had a histopathologic diagnosis. Of 15 patients, 7 had acute osteomyelitis and 8 had chronic osteomyelitis or inflammatory spondylitis. FDG-PET yielded true-positive results in all 15 patients, whereas bone scintigraphy performed in 11 patients yielded 10 true-positive results and 1 false-negative result. Thus, FDG-PET was clearly superior to bone scintigraphy for the diagnosis of bone infection. Follow-up FDG-PET scans were performed in 2 patients and showed normalization of FDG uptake correlating well with clinical data. The limitation of FDG-PET described in this study was its inability to differentiate between postsurgical reactive changes and further infection during early postoperative follow-up.

As mentioned previously, when discussing bone infections, the important issue that needs to be worked out is differentiation between postsurgical inflammation (normal healing process) and infection. Koort and colleagues [29] conducted an experimental study to evaluate whether FDG-PET can differentiate between normal bone healing compared with the healing of bone with local osteomyelitis. A localized osteomyelitis model of the rabbit tibia was created, and two groups were created (osteomyelitis group [n = 8] and normal inflammation group [n = 8]). In the normal inflammation group, uncomplicated bone healing was associated with an initial increase in FDG uptake at 3 weeks, which subsequently returned to normal by 6 weeks. Conversely, in the osteomyelitis group, localized infection resulted in intense continuous uptake of FDG. Therefore, FDG-PET was clearly beneficial in the postsurgical follow-up. Similarly, FDG-PET is also expected to be beneficial in differentiating between infection and sterile inflammation or sterile stress fractures in patients with metallic implants and prostheses.

Prosthesis infection

Superimposed infection in prosthetic implants is a common occurrence and needs to be detected at the earliest possible point so that appropriate intervention can be instituted. A significant long-term complication of hip arthroplasty is aseptic loosening, which can even lead to prostheses reimplantation. Aseptic loosening and superimposed infections are sometimes difficult to differentiate. Various nuclear medicine techniques, such as leukocyte scans, sulfur colloid bone marrow scans, bone scintigraphy, and FDG-PET scans, have been studied to differentiate between these two conditions [30–32]. FDG-PET has not been extensively studied for this purpose but holds great future promise. FDG-PET has shown mixed results to date, but more studies are needed before a definite conclusion can be made.

Zhuang and coworkers [33] followed two groups of patients with arthroplasty to assess the patterns and time course of FDG accumulation after total hip replacement over an extended period. In first group, 9 patients were investigated prospectively with PET scans at 3, 6, and 12 months after arthroplasty. The second group involved a retrospective analysis of 18 patients with a history of 21 hip arthroplasties who had undergone PET for the evaluation of possible malignant disorders but were asymptomatic for arthroplasty. The authors demonstrated increased FDG uptake around the femoral head or neck portion of the prosthesis that extended to the soft tissues surrounding the femur in all 9 patients in the first group. In second group of asymptomatic patients, 81% (17 of 21) showed increased FDG uptake around the femoral head or neck portion of the prosthesis. The average time interval between the arthroplasty and FDG-PET scan in these patients was 71.3 months. In only 4 (19%) of 21 prostheses was no abnormally increased FDG uptake seen around the prostheses or adjacent sites. The average time interval in these patients was 114.8 months. The authors concluded that after hip arthroplasty, nonspecific increased FDG uptake around the head or neck of the prosthesis persists for many years, even in patients without any complications.

FDG uptake is also increased in sterile inflammation secondary to surgery. Chacko and coworkers [34] found that quantification of FDG uptake is not always a good parameter for evaluation of FDG-PET when characterizing infections. They studied the location and intensity of FDG uptake in 41 total hip arthroplasties from 32 patients with a complete clinical follow-up. Twelve patients had periprosthetic infection, and 11 of these displayed moderately increased tracer uptake along the interface between the bone and the prosthesis. In contrast, images from sterile loose hip prostheses revealed intense uptake around the head or neck of the prosthesis with SUVs as high as 7. These investigators concluded that the intensity of increased FDG uptake is less important than the location of the increased FDG uptake when FDG-PET is used to diagnose periprosthetic infection in patients with hip arthroplasty.

Atherosclerosis

Atherosclerosis is the leading cause of illness and death in the United States. Atherosclerosis is a slow progressive disease that may start in childhood [35,36]. It affects chiefly the aorta, arteries of the brain, heart, kidneys, and arms and legs. Inflammation is well documented in the literature as an integral part of atherosclerosis [37,38]. Studies from the laboratory have shown that there is no measurable FDG uptake in the normal vessel wall but that inflammatory cells, predominantly macrophages, take up FDG in atherosclerotic plaques [39]. Thus, as a functional imaging modality, FDG-PET can detect and localize inflammatory changes in the arterial wall representing early stages of atherosclerosis [40]. In addition, FDG-PET can be used in quantifying the degree of atherosclerosis by using SUVs.

Early detection of therapy response in coronary atherosclerosis is of considerable importance because it can direct one to intervene at the earliest possible point, if needed. Baller and colleagues [41] demonstrated improvement in coronary flow reserve as demonstrated by PET after 6 months of cholesterol-lowering therapy in patients with early stages of coronary atherosclerosis. A total of 23 consecutive patients in the early stages of coronary atherosclerosis were investigated. All patients underwent myocardial blood flow measurement with N-13 ammonia PET at rest and under dipyridamole stress before and after lipid-lowering therapy. Maximal coronary flow increased significantly from 182 ± 36 mL/min $\times$ 100 g to 238 ± 58 mL/min $\times$ 100 g ($P < .001$) after a 6-month treatment with simvastatin. Further studies are needed for this purpose. The authors concluded that PET could assess the effects of cholesterol-lowering therapy noninvasively.

Others

There are a few isolated case studies and case reports regarding the role of PET in evaluation of the treatment response in various inflammatory or infectious diseases. Kotilainen and colleagues [42] reported the case of 41-year-old patient with Riedel's thyroiditis, in whom FDG-PET demonstrated intensive FDG uptake in both lobes of the thyroid gland as an indication of severe inflammation. On follow-up of corticosteroid treatment after 2 weeks, an FDG-PET scan showed a 60% decrease in the uptake of FDG in the thyroid. Drieskens and coworkers [43] reported a case of multifocal fibrosclerosis manifesting as retroperitoneal fibrosis and Riedel's thyroiditis. There was increased FDG uptake in the abdomen surrounding the aorta and in the thyroid, which normalized after 4 weeks of steroid therapy. The authors proposed that FDG-PET may help to diagnose and evaluate the treatment response in patients with multifocal fibrosclerosis.

Tsuyuguchi and colleagues [44] evaluated FDG-PET and C11-methionine PET before and after treatment in four patients with a brain abscess. The baseline PET scan showed uptake of both tracers in the brain abscess. After treatment, the lesion area became small on enhancement with CT or MRI, and PET studies showed a reduced lesion size with decreased radiotracer uptake. The authors concluded that PET was useful in detecting the inflammatory lesion and assessing the clinical effects of antibiotic treatment on brain abscesses.

Scheid and coworkers [45] performed serial MRI and FDG-PET scans in a patient with anti-Ma2-positive paraneoplastic limbic encephalitis. They found focal tracer accumulation in the left medial temporal lobe, which increased during the first 9 months of follow-up with FDG-PET. MRI findings showing a hyperintense signal change in the left medial temporal lobe remained unchanged over time.

Moosig and colleagues [46] evaluated the role of FDG-PET in 13 untreated patients with active polymyalgia rheumatica. Follow-up PET scans were analyzed in 8 patients while they were in clinical remission. By visual evaluation, 12 of the 13 patients showed increased tracer uptake in the aorta or its major branches. By quantitative analysis, FDG uptake was significantly increased in polymyalgia rheumatica. In the 8 patients who underwent follow-up PET, the index declined substantially after clinical remission. In this study, FDG uptake was significantly correlated with serologic markers of inflammation, such as C-reactive protein, ESR, and platelet counts.

Bleeker-Rovers and coworkers [47] studied FDG-PET scans in three patients with adult polycystic kidney diseases with suspicion of renal or hepatic cyst infection. Seven PET scans were performed in three patients. Of these three patients, two had a follow-up PET scan. In one patient, the follow-up FDG-PET scan was normal after 6 weeks of antibiotic treatment for hepatic cyst infection.

In an experimental animal study, Wyss and colleagues [48] evaluated the influence of ceftriaxone treatment on FDG uptake in soft tissue infections in rats. Three PET scans were performed in each of two groups (four treated animals and four nontreated animals) on days 3, 5, and 6 after inoculation of the infection. Additional autoradiography was performed in four animals on day 7 and in three animals on day 11. The difference in FDG uptake on day 5 between the two groups was significant, although it was not significant on other days. Further evaluation is necessary to delineate the role of FDG-PET in soft tissue infections.

Win and coworkers [49] reported a case of *Pneumocystis carinii* pneumonia in a 26-year-old man with moderate to severe leukopenia. FDG-PET demonstrated acute lung changes, which disappeared on the follow-up scan after treatment. The authors proposed that FDG-PET might prove useful in the diagnosis and evaluation of the treatment response in patients with *Pneumocystis carinii* pneumonia.

Summary

There is a definite role for FDG-PET in the diagnosis and evaluation of the treatment response and disease activity in patients with vasculitis. Although the data for FDG-PET are limited in other inflammatory or infectious diseases, the results are encouraging and PET seems to have a promising future role in the follow-up of inflammatory or infectious diseases.

References

[1] Kumar R, Nadig MR, Chauhan A. Positron emission tomography: clinical applications in oncology. Part 1. Expert Rev Anticancer Ther 2005;5:1079–94.

[2] Kostakoglu L, Agress Jr H, Goldsmith SJ. Clinical role of FDG PET in evaluation of cancer patients. Radiographics 2003;23:315–40.

[3] Kumar R, Bhargava P, Bozkurt MF, et al. Positron emission tomography imaging in evaluation of cancer patients. Indian J Cancer 2003;40:87–100.

[4] Avril N, Sassen S, Schmalfeldt B, et al. Prediction of response to neoadjuvant chemotherapy by sequential F-18-fluorodeoxyglucose positron emission tomography in patients with advanced-stage ovarian cancer. J Clin Oncol 2005;23:7445–53.

[5] Kumar R, Xiu Y, Potenta S, et al. 18F-FDG PET for evaluation of the treatment response in patients with gastrointestinal tract lymphomas. J Nucl Med 2004;45:1796–803.

[6] Dose Schwarz J, Bader M, Jenicke L, et al. Early prediction of response to chemotherapy in metastatic breast cancer using sequential 18F-FDG PET. J Nucl Med 2005;46:1144–50.

[7] Theron J, Tyler JL. Takayasu's arteritis of the aortic arch: endovascular treatment and correlation with positron emission tomography. AJNR Am J Neuroradiol 1987;8:621–6.

[8] Zhuang H, Pourdehnad M, Lambright ES, et al. Dual time point 18F-FDG PET imaging for differentiating malignant from inflammatory processes. J Nucl Med 2001;42:1412–7.

[9] Kumar R, Loving VA, Chauhan A, et al. Potential of dual-time-point imaging to improve breast cancer diagnosis with (18)F-FDG PET. J Nucl Med 2005;46:1819–24.

[10] Hustinx R, Smith RJ, Benard F, et al. Dual time point fluorine-18 fluorodeoxyglucose positron emission tomography: a potential method to

differentiate malignancy from inflammation and normal tissue in the head and neck. Eur J Nucl Med 1999;26:1345–8.

[11] Hara M, Goodman PC, Leder RA. FDG-PET finding in early-phase Takayasu arteritis. J Comput Assist Tomogr 1999;23:16–8.

[12] Meller J, Grabbe E, Becker W, et al. Value of F-18FDG hybrid camera PET and MRI in early Takayasu aortitis. Eur Radiol 2003;13:400–5.

[13] Brodmann M, Lipp RW, Passath A, et al. The role of 2-F-18-fluoro-2-deoxy-D-glucose positron emission tomography in the diagnosis of giant cell arteritis of the temporal arteries. Rheumatology (Oxford) 2004;43:241–2.

[14] Balan K, Voutnis D, Groves A. Discordant uptake of F-18FDG and In-111WBC in systemic vasculitis. Clin Nucl Med 2003;28:485–6.

[15] Derdelinckx I, Maes A, Bogaert J, et al. Positron emission tomography scan in the diagnosis and follow-up of aortitis of the thoracic aorta. Acta Cardiol 2000;55:193–5.

[16] Turlakow A, Yeung HW, Pui J, et al. Fludeoxyglucose positron emission tomography in the diagnosis of giant cell arteritis. Arch Intern Med 2001;161:1003–7.

[17] Meller J, Strutz F, Siefker U, et al. Early diagnosis and follow-up of aortitis with [(18)F]FDG PET and MRI. Eur J Nucl Med Mol Imaging 2003;30:730–6.

[18] Moreno D, Yuste JR, Rodriguez M, et al. Positron emission tomography use in the diagnosis and follow up of Takayasu's arteritis. Ann Rheum Dis 2005;64:1091–3.

[19] Bleeker-Rovers CP, Bredie SJ, van der Meer JW, et al. F-18-fluorodeoxyglucose positron emission tomography in diagnosis and follow-up of patients with different types of vasculitis. Neth J Med 2003;61:323–9.

[20] Bleeker-Rovers CP, Bredie SJ, van der Meer JW, et al. Fluorine 18 fluorodeoxyglucose positron emission tomography in the diagnosis and follow-up of three patients with vasculitis. Am J Med 2004;116:50–3.

[21] de Leeuw K, Bijl M, Jager PL. Additional value of positron emission tomography in diagnosis and follow-up of patients with large vessel vasculitides. Clin Exp Rheumatol 2004;22(Suppl):S21–6.

[22] Webb M, Chambers A, Al-Nahhas A, et al. The role of 18F-FDG PET in characterising disease activity in Takayasu arteritis. Eur J Nucl Med Mol Imaging 2004;31:627–34.

[23] Andrews J, Al-Nahhas A, Pennell DJ, et al. Non-invasive imaging in the diagnosis and management of Takayasu's arteritis. Ann Rheum Dis 2004;63:995–1000.

[24] Scheel AK, Meller J, Vosshenrich R, et al. Diagnosis and follow up of aortitis in the elderly. Ann Rheum Dis 2004;63:1507–10.

[25] De Winter F, Van de Wiele C, Vogelaers D, et al. Fluorine-18 fluorodeoxyglucose-positron emission tomography: a highly accurate imaging modality for the diagnosis of chronic musculoskeletal infections. J Bone Joint Surg Am 2001;83:651–60.

[26] Meller J, Koster G, Liersch T, et al. Chronic bacterial osteomyelitis: prospective comparison of F-18-FDG imaging with a dual-head coincidence camera and In-111-labelled autologous leucocyte scintigraphy. Eur J Nucl Med 2002;29:53–60.

[27] Robiller FC, Stumpe KDM, Kossmann T, et al. Chronic osteomyelitis of the femur: value of PET imaging. Eur Radiol 2000;10:855–8.

[28] Kalicke T, Schmitz A, Risse JH, et al. Fluorine-18 fluorodeoxyglucose PET in infectious bone diseases: results of histologically confirmed cases. Eur J Nucl Med 2000;27:524–8.

[29] Koort JK, Makinen TJ, Knuuti J, et al. Comparative 18F-FDG PET of experimental Staphylococcus aureus osteomyelitis and normal bone healing. J Nucl Med 2004;45:1406–11.

[30] El Espera I, Blondet C, Moullart V, et al. The usefulness of 99mTc sulfur colloid bone marrow scintigraphy combined with 111In leucocyte scintigraphy in prosthetic joint infection. Nucl Med Commun 2004;25:171–5.

[31] Joseph TN, Mujtaba M, Chen AL, et al. Efficacy of combined technetium-99m sulfur colloid/indium-111 leukocyte scans to detect infected total hip and knee arthroplasties. J Arthroplasty 2001;16:753–8.

[32] Love C, Marwin SE, Tomas MB, et al. Diagnosing infection in the failed joint replacement: a comparison of coincidence detection 18F-FDG and 111In-labeled leukocyte/99mTc-sulfur colloid marrow imaging. J Nucl Med 2004;45:1864–71.

[33] Zhuang H, Chacko TK, Hickeson M, et al. Persistent non-specific FDG uptake on PET imaging following hip arthroplasty. Eur J Nucl Med Mol Imaging 2002;29:1328–33.

[34] Chacko TK, Zhuang H, Stevenson K, et al. The importance of the location of fluorodeoxyglucose uptake in periprosthetic infection in painful hip prostheses. Nucl Med Commun 2002;23:851–5.

[35] Kortelainen ML. Adiposity, cardiac size and precursors of coronary atherosclerosis in 5 to 15-year-old children: a retrospective study of 210 violent deaths. Int J Obes Relat Metab Disord 1997;21:691–7.

[36] Daniels SR. Cardiovascular disease risk factors and atherosclerosis in children and adolescents. Curr Atheroscler Rep 2001;3:479–85.

[37] Andrews J, Al-Nahhas A, Pennell D, et al. Non-invasive imaging in the diagnosis and management of Takayasu's arteritis. Ann Rheum Dis 2004;63:995–1000.

[38] Ben-Haim S, Kupzov E, Tamir A, et al. Evaluation of 18F-FDG uptake and arterial wall calcifications using 18F-FDG PET/CT. J Nucl Med 2004;45:1816–21.

[39] El-Haddad G, Zhuang H, Gupta N, et al. Evolving

role of positron emission tomography in the management of patients with inflammatory and other benign disorders. Semin Nucl Med 2004; 34:313–29.

[40] Rudd JH, Warburton EA, Fryer TD, et al. Imaging atherosclerotic plaque inflammation with [^{18}F]-fluorodeoxyglucose positron emission tomography. Circulation 2002;105:2708–11.

[41] Baller D, Notohamiprodjo G, Gleichmann U, et al. Improvement in coronary flow reserve determined by positron emission tomography after 6 months of cholesterol-lowering therapy in patients with early stages of coronary atherosclerosis. Circulation 1999;99:2871–5.

[42] Kotilainen P, Airas L, Kojo T, et al. Positron emission tomography as an aid in the diagnosis and follow-up of Riedel's thyroiditis. Eur J Intern Med 2004;15:186–9.

[43] Drieskens O, Blockmans D, Van den Bruel A, et al. Riedel's thyroiditis and retroperitoneal fibrosis in multifocal fibrosclerosis: positron emission tomographic findings. Clin Nucl Med 2002; 27:413–5.

[44] Tsuyuguchi N, Sunada I, Ohata K, et al. Evaluation of treatment effects in brain abscess with positron emission tomography: comparison of fluorine-18-fluorodeoxyglucose and carbon-11-methionine. Ann Nucl Med 2003;17:47–51.

[45] Scheid R, Lincke T, Voltz R, et al. Serial 18F-fluoro-2-deoxy-D-glucose positron emission tomography and magnetic resonance imaging of paraneoplastic limbic encephalitis. Arch Neurol 2004;61:1785–9.

[46] Moosig F, Czech N, Mehl C, et al. Correlation between 18-fluorodeoxyglucose accumulation in large vessels and serological markers of inflammation in polymyalgia rheumatica: a quantitative PET study. Ann Rheum Dis 2004;63:870–3.

[47] Bleeker-Rovers CP, de Sevaux RG, van Hamersvelt HW, et al. Diagnosis of renal and hepatic cyst infections by 18-F-fluorodeoxyglucose positron emission tomography in autosomal dominant polycystic kidney disease. Am J Kidney Dis 2003; 41:E18–21.

[48] Wyss MT, Honer M, Spath N, et al. Influence of ceftriaxone treatment on FDG uptake—an in vivo [18F]-fluorodeoxyglucose imaging study in soft tissue infections in rats. Nucl Med Biol 2004; 31:875–82.

[49] Win Z, Todd J, Al-Nahhas A. FDG-PET imaging in Pneumocystis carinii pneumonia. Clin Nucl Med 2005;30:690–1.

ELSEVIER
SAUNDERS

POSITRON
EMISSION
TOMOGRAPHY

PET Clin 1 (2006) 199–202

Index

Note: Page numbers of article titles are in **boldface** type.

A

Abdominal abscess, fever of unknown origin in, 165
Abscess
    abdominal, fever of unknown origin in, 165
    brain, 196
Adenopathy, hilar, in sarcoidosis, 142
American Association of Nuclear Medicine, vasculitis
  scan protocols of, 182
Angiography, magnetic resonance, in vasculitis,
  193–194
Antigranulocyte antibody scintigraphy
    in inflammatory bowel disease, 154
    in osteomyelitis, 114–115, 117–118
Aortitis, PET in, 192–194
Arteritis
    giant cell. *See* Giant cell arteritis.
    Takayasu's. *See* Takayasu's arteritis.
Arthritis
    psoriatic, PET in, 132
    rheumatoid. *See* Rheumatoid arthritis.
Arthroplasty, infection in, **99–106**
    PET in
        accuracy of, 100–102
        CT with, 103
        in allograft evaluation, 103–104
        in treatment assessment, 194–195
        suboptimal results in, 102–103
Atherosclerosis, PET in, 182–184, 195

B

Bone
    healing of, FDG uptake in, 112–114
    infections of. *See* Osteomyelitis.
Bone graft, in arthroplasty, 103
Brain
    abscess of, 196
    sarcoidosis of, 149

C

Cancer
    fever of unknown origin in, 164–165
    PET in, versus inflammation, 182, 192
Charcot foot. *See* Diabetic foot.
Coincidence PET camera
    in arthroplasty infections, 102–103
    in osteomyelitis, 115–116
Colitis, ulcerative. *See* Inflammatory bowel disease.
Collagen vascular diseases, fever of unknown origin
  in, 165
Computed tomography
    in fever of unknown origin, 168
    in rheumatoid arthritis, 134–135
    in sarcoidosis, 142, 145
    PET combined with. *See* PET/CT.
Crohn's disease. *See* Inflammatory bowel disease.
CT. *See* Computed tomography.

D

Diabetic foot, **123–130**
    epidemiology of, 124
    pathophysiology of, 124
    PET in, 125–128
    radiography in, 124
    scintigraphy in, 124–125
Dual-headed coincidence PET camera, in
  osteomyelitis, 115–116

E

EF5 [2-(2-nitro-1[H]-imidazol-1-yl)-
  N-(2,2,3,3,3-pentafluoropropyl)-acetamide],
  in diabetic foot, 128
European Association of Nuclear Medicine, vasculitis
  scan protocols of, 182

pet.theclinics.com   doi:10.1016/S1556-8598(06)00031-9

F

FDG. *See* [^{18}F]-Fluorodeoxyglucose.
Fever of unknown origin, **163–177**
  causes of, 164–165
  computed tomography in, 168
  definition of, 164
  differential diagnosis of, 164–165
  PET in, 166–173
    basis for, 166
    limitations of, 171
    literature review of, 171–173
    mechanism of action of, 166
    versus anatomic imaging, 167–171
    versus other nuclear medicine techniques,
      166–167
  radiography in, 165
  scintigraphy in, 165–166
  subcategories of, 164
Fibrosclerosis, multifocal, 196
[^{18}F]-Fluorodeoxyglucose
  biodistribution of, 109–110
  in arthritis, **131–139**
  in arthroplasty infections, **99–106**
  in diabetic foot, **123–130**
  in fever of unknown origin, **163–177**
  in inflammatory bowel disease, **153–162**
  in large vessel vasculitis, **179–189**
  in osteomyelitis, **107–121**
  in sarcoidosis, **141–152**
  in therapy response assessment, **191–198**
  uptake of. *See also specific disorders.*
    in inflammatory cells, 110–111
    physiology of, 109, 192
[^{18}F]-Fluoro-methyl-tyrosine, in PET, in
  sarcoidosis, 148
Foot
  diabetic. *See* Diabetic foot.
  rheumatoid arthritis of, 133
Fractures, healing of, FDG uptake in, 112–114

G

Gallium-67, in scintigraphy
  in fever of unknown origin, 167
  in sarcoidosis, 142–145, 149
Gallium-68, in scintigraphy, in diabetic foot, 127–128
Giant cell arteritis
  clinical features of, 181
  diagnosis of, 181–182
  epidemiology of, 181
  fever of unknown origin in, 165
  magnetic resonance imaging in, 184
  pathophysiology of, 180–181
  PET in, 182–185, 192–194
Glucose, levels of, FDG uptake and, 111–112,
  126–127

Glucose transporters (GLUTs), FDG uptake by, 110
GLUTs (glucose transporters), FDG uptake by, 110
Granulocytes, FDG uptake by, 110
Granulomas, in sarcoidosis, 142
Growth factors, in bone healing, 112

H

Hand, rheumatoid arthritis of, 133
Healing, bone, FDG uptake in, 112–114
Heart, sarcoidosis of, 148–149
Hematogenous osteomyelitis, 108
Hilar adenopathy, in sarcoidosis, 142
Hip arthroplasty, infection in, **99–106**, 195
Human immunodeficiency virus infection, fever of
  unknown origin in, 164, 166
Hyperglycemia, FDG uptake and, 126–127
Hyperinsulinemia, FDG uptake in, 112

I

Immunoglobulin, nonspecific, in scintigraphy, in
  inflammatory bowel disease, 154
Indium-111, in scintigraphy
  in diabetic foot, 124
  in inflammatory bowel disease, 155
  in sarcoidosis, 144
Infection and inflammation
  arthritis, **131–139**
  diabetic foot, 109, **123–130**
  fever of unknown origin, **163–177**
  in arthroplasty, **99–106**, 194–195
  inflammatory bowel disease, **153–162**
  large vessel vasculitis, **179–189**, 192–194
  osteomyelitis. *See* Osteomyelitis.
  sarcoidosis, **141–152**
  therapy response assessment in, **191–198**
Inflammation. *See* Infection and inflammation.
Inflammatory bowel disease, **153–162**
  pathophysiology of, 154–156
  PET in, 156–158
  radiopharmaceuticals for, 154–156
Insulin levels, FDG uptake and, 112

J

Juvenile rheumatoid arthritis, fever of unknown origin
  in, 165

K

Kidney, polycystic disease of, PET in, 196
Knee
  arthroplasty of, infection in, **99–106**
  rheumatoid arthritis of, 133